The Thyroid Sourcebook for Women

Also by M. Sara Rosenthal:

The Thyroid Sourcebook, 3rd edition

The Gynecological Sourcebook, 3rd edition

The Pregnancy Sourcebook, 3rd edition

The Fertility Sourcebook, 3rd edition

The Breastfeeding Sourcebook, 2nd edition

The Breast Sourcebook, 2nd edition

The Gastrointestinal Sourcebook

The Type 2 Diabetic Woman

Managing Your Diabetes:
The Only Complete Guide to Type 2 Diabetes for Canadians

Managing Diabetes for Women:
The Only Canadian Women's Guide to Type 2 Diabetes

The Thyroid Sourcebook for Women

M. Sara Rosenthal

Foreword by Kelly R. Hale,
Founder/President,
American Foundation of Thyroid Patients

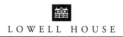

LOWELL HOUSE

LOS ANGELES

NTC/Contemporary Publishing Group

The purpose of this book is to educate. It is sold with the understanding that the author and publisher shall have neither liability nor responsibility for any injury caused or alleged to be caused directly or indirectly by the information contained in this book. While every effort has been made to ensure its accuracy, the book's contents should not be construed as medical advice. Each person's health needs are unique. To obtain recommendations appropriate to your particular situation, please consult a qualified health-care provider.

Library of Congress Cataloging-in-Publication Data

Rosenthal, M. Sara.
    The thyroid sourcebook for women / M. Sara Rosenthal ; foreword by Kelly Hale.
      p.   cm.
    Includes bibliographical references and index.
    ISBN 0-7373-0264-X
    1. Thyroid gland—Diseases Popular works. 2. Women—Diseases Popular works. I. Title.
    RC655.R673 1999
    616.4'4'0082—dc21   99-39865
                                                         CIP

Cover design by Monica Baziuk
Design by Jack Lanning

Published by Lowell House
A division of NTC/Contemporary Publishing Group, Inc.
4255 West Touhy Avenue, Lincolnwood, Illinois 60712, U.S.A.
Copyright © 1999 by M. Sara Rosenthal
Printed in the United States of America
International Standard Book Number: 0-7373-0264-X
    01 02 03 04 DOC   18 17 16 15 14 13 12 11 10 9 8 7 6 5

For my mother, Naomi

Contents

Foreword

Sara Rosenthal has done it again! Being a thyroid patient herself, she brings much needed insight and a little humor to a very nonglamorous disease.

If you are a woman who is newly diagnosed with a thyroid disorder, this book will serve as your "bible." Read it cover to cover. If you are a "veteran" thyroid patient, you may choose to use it as a reference when questions arise. Either way, it is an invaluable tool that no woman should be without. I say this because thyroid disease is estimated to affect some twenty-one million Americans (80 percent are women), and half of those twenty-one million are undiagnosed or misdiagnosed. The statistics only increase for women as we age; many of us will indeed develop a thyroid condition at some point in our lifetime.

In fact, this book should be shared with family members and friends so that they can better understand your moods, energy levels (or lack thereof!), and gain the knowledge to provide understanding and moral support. In addition, it will increase awareness that thyroid disease has familial tendencies; if you should happen to be male, then you are not immune to thyroid disease, either!

More than likely, most of us reading this book will deal with thyroid disease in some form or fashion for the remainder of our lives, as well as juggle a myriad of female hormone issues at any given stage of life.

Considering that thyroid disease is a lifelong condition, it is essential that we become better educated about our health condition while becoming more savvy medical consumers given the countless health-care alternatives we face today.

It is my suggestion that you keep this book close at hand. It will be there for you, the hyperthyroid patient, wide awake at 4:00 A.M., when no one else will be; and for you, the hypothyroid patient, as you drag yourself out of bed wondering if you will ever have enough energy to keep up with your life "as you knew it before," and who remembers reading about combination therapy. Take this book with you when you see your doctor and discuss the potential benefits mentioned herein.

This book provides the keys to unlock the "mysteries and myths" surrounding thyroid disease and women. Ms. Rosenthal provides easy-to-understand information, and I am particularly fond of the cross-reference annotations.

To thyroid patients everywhere—good reading and good health!

        Kelly R. Hale,
        Founder/President,
        American Foundation of Thyroid Patients
        "Empowerment through Education and Support"

Acknowledgments

I wish to thank the following people, whose expertise and dedication as medical advisers on previous works helped to lay so much of the groundwork for this book:

Robert Volpe, M.D., F.R.C.P., F.A.C.P.
Suzanne Pratt, M.D., F.A.C.O.G.
Masood Khathamee, M.D., F.A.C.O.G.
Gillian Arsenault, M.D., C.C.F.P., I.B.L.C., F.R.C.P.
Pamela Craig, M.D., F.A.C.S., Ph.D.
James McSherry, M.B., Ch.B., F.C.F.P., F.R.C.G.P.,
    F.A.A.F.P., F.A.B.M.P.
Gary May, M.D., F.R.C.P.
Susan George, M.D., F.R.C.P., F.A.C.P.
Irving B. Rosen, M.D., F.R.C.S., F.A.C.S.
Matthew Lazar, M.D., F.R.C.P., F.A.C.P.
Debra Lander, M.D., F.R.C.P.

I'd also like to thank Kelly Hale, Founder/President, American Foundation of Thyroid Patients, for her immediate and unwavering support of this venture.

William Harvey, Ph.D, LL.B., Director, University of Toronto Joint Centre for Bioethics, whose devotion to bioethics has inspired me, continues to support my work, and makes it possible for me to have the courage to question and challenge issues in health care and medical ethics. Irving Rootman, Ph.D., Director, University of Toronto Centre for Health Promotion, continues to encourage my interest in primary prevention and health promotion issues. Helen Lenskyj, Ph.D., Professor, Department of Sociology and Equity Studies, Ontario Institute for Studies in Education/University of Toronto, and Laura M. Purdy, Ph.D., Department of Philosophy, University of Toronto, and Bioethicist, University of Toronto Joint Centre for Bioethics, have been central figures in my understanding of the complexities of women's health issues and feminist bioethics.

Larissa Kostoff, my editoral assistant, worked very hard to make this book come to fruition. Bud Sperry at Lowell House has been patient and supportive as always. Special thanks to the production team, Maria Magallanes and Jama Carter.

And finally, I continue to appreciate the support that comes from my friends and family members.

Introduction

A Woman's Disease

The inspiration to write about thyroid disease came from the women in my family. From my great-grandmother who developed a goiter in the 1930s. From my grandmother who developed Graves' disease in 1940 with her first pregnancy at twenty-four, had her thyroid removed, and was not given any subsequent medication because her doctor said she "didn't need it." From my mother, who developed Graves' disease in 1981, watched in dismay as her eyes bulged out like *her* mother's, and read through stacks of complicated medical texts to try to find out more about her illness. From my aunt, who became severely hypothyroid in her late thirties, and her daughter, who developed thyroid cancer at age twenty. And from my older sister, who in 1991 had to beg her family doctor for a thyroid test on her thirtieth birthday because thyroid disorders "run in the family." Her doctor reluctantly ordered the test and was surprised to find out that my sister had Graves' disease, too.

My family's thyroid heritage is statistically not remarkable. In 1983, when I turned twenty, my family's "legacy" was passed down to me as well: I was diagnosed with thyroid cancer. Within a short span of months, my thyroid gland and the lymph nodes on the right side of my neck were surgically removed. I was then required to drink radioactive iodine a couple of times from a lead container. In my final treatment stage, every morning for an entire month I visited a hospital basement for external radiation therapy. On my twenty-first birthday, I was given the "all clear." But I was never given any information about what I had gone through and continue to live with.

I had to rely on relatives and friends of friends who were doctors for basic "What's a thyroid?" information. I flirted with the interns so that I could be privy to juicy facts and tidbits on the thyroid gland, and was reduced to "eavesdropping" on my surgeon (*while* he was examining me) as he outlined my history and prognosis to the troupe of medical students with him on his "rounds." I rudely interrupted his "lecture" one day and dared to ask him a question. Everyone looked surprised, and one student asked me if I was "in sciences." Patients should be seen and not heard was the message.

Today, as I look back on my experience, I understand the feminist adage: "The personal is political." By this I mean that within one woman's story about her feelings and struggles with her body lies the story of all women's feelings and struggles with their bodies. And within *that* story lies the social history of women's health. Women's struggles with thyroid disease tell the story of how women are treated in the health-care system. Since the publication of my first book on thyroid disease, *The Thyroid Sourcebook,* I have spoken to women all over North America and the United Kingdom about their experiences with this disease and have come to view thyroid disease as a "test case" for women's general health. Dr. Laura Purdy, a feminist philosopher and bioethicist has this to say about women's health:

> It hardly needs saying that despite considerable progress for
> women in recent years, men—mostly white, middle-class,
> heterosexual men—still in charge, both in society generally and in
> the medical profession, and, consciously or subconsciously,
> choose social arrangements that reflect their perceived interests.
> Worse still, individual practitioners may still be gripped by
> common sexist—even misogynist—attitudes for which medical
> education currently provides no antidote . . . (For example,) how
> could we have been so oblivious to the gender differences in
> physician–patient relationships, differences that lead doctors to

suppose that women need tranquilizers when the same symptoms in a man suggest a heart workup. (Purdy 1996: 2–3)

But what Dr. Purdy points out in this quote is no different than what women have been saying to me for years about their experiences with thyroid disease: many are ignored or misdiagnosed with stress-related or psychiatric disorders; many are unable to obtain adequate information from their doctors about thyroid disease; many are abused and "infantilized" (i.e., treated like children) by their physicians.

When my first book on thyroid disease was published in 1993, it was exactly ten years after my own thyroid surgery and treatment. I wasn't sure how people were going to respond to medical information provided in such plain, nontechnical language. As a journalist and someone who had experienced every imaginable thyroid test and treatment, I took up the task, and then, my readers continued to pass on *The Thyroid Sourcebook* torch. Now in its third revised edition, it was clear that a thyroid book that focused solely on women was much needed. When I wrote *The Thyroid Sourcebook,* I wrote the book I wish *I* had when I was diagnosed. The book you have in your hands is the book I need now, as my reproductive organs mature and I approach my forties and fifties.

Over thirteen million people in the United States and Canada alone suffer from thyroid disorders—and thyroid disorders occur at least ten times more frequently in women. Hypothyroidism affects at least 8 percent of all women over age sixty-five. But new evidence from the National Cancer Institute reveals that people who were exposed as children to fallout from nuclear testing during the 1950s and early 1960s may be more at risk for thyroid disorders or thyroid cancer as adults. Those living in midwestern North America are particularly at risk.

As a woman dealing with thyroid disease, you are also dealing with a myriad of other health concerns. This book is designed to help you make informed choices about health care. "Informed consent" is a guiding principle for medical practitioners and researchers. It means that in order for someone to make an informed decision, there must be full disclosure of all risks and benefits; that person must completely understand what's being explained; that person must be fully competent; and that person must feel free to say "yes" or "no" according to his or her own wishes, values, and "gut feeling" without any coercion or coaxing.

Given the highly technical nature of many of the tests and procedures discussed in this book, and the fact that many drugs have not been tested on women, is it even reasonable to expect that women *can* make informed decisions?

Most bioethicists agree that informed consent is an oxymoron, like "jumbo shrimp"; the two ideas are incompatible. Because to be truly informed when it comes to many medical procedures (thyroid or otherwise), it's often not good enough to know "what time it is"; you need to know how to build a watch. The problem with "informed consent" is that unless *you* are a doctor, how informed can you really become?

There are also problems concerning whose interests are being served by certain procedures. And too often, if you decline a particular treatment you're considered to be uninformed while many doctors will treat your "consent" to a procedure as proof that you *are* informed—when, in fact, you are not.

So whenever you consent to any kind of medical test, procedure, or treatment, here are all the things your doctor should disclose to you:

- A description of the test, procedure, or treatment and its expected effects (e.g., duration of hospital stay, expected time of recovery, restrictions on daily activities, scars).
- Information about relevant alternative options and their expected benefits and relevant risks.
- An explanation of the consequences of declining or delaying treatment.

Your doctor should also give you an opportunity to ask questions—and should be available to answer them. Here are all the questions you must ask yourself:

1. Do *you* understand the information relevant to your decision, and do you appreciate the reasonably foreseeable

consequences of your decision or *lack* of decision? This is what is known as your *capacity* to consent to procedures.

2. Do you understand what is being disclosed, and can you make your decision based on this information?

3. Are you being allowed to make your decision free of any undue influences? (For example, are you in pain? Is information being distorted or omitted? Are you being sedated?) This is what is known as *voluntariness;* involuntary consent means, of course, that you have not consented to a procedure.

If you answered "no" to any of these questions, you are probably not being given adequate information, or you are in no condition to make a decision about your health.

There are also different medical personalities of doctors, which will affect how information is being disclosed to you. For example, a "paternalistic" doctor usually makes the decision for you or strongly suggests an approach. An "informative" doctor presents, in theory, enough information for you to make your own choice, but because your doctor knows more than you do, it may be unrealistic for you to actually make your own decision.

On that note, I leave it to you to use this book to help yourself better understand thyroid disease and how your thyroid condition will affect your health-care decisions throughout your life. Please accept this second thyroid book as the "second torch." Pass it on to another woman who is suffering not so much from thyroid disease, but from *no information* about *her* thyroid disease.

CHAPTER 1

All About Eve— And the Thyroid Gland

At least 1 in 10 women can expect to suffer from some sort of thyroid disorder during her lifetime. Whether thyroid disorders strike at puberty, during peak reproductive years, during or after pregnancy, around menopause, or after age sixty, a woman's body is uniquely—and dramatically—affected. The most common thyroid disease (Graves' disease, which causes an overactive thyroid gland) occurs *fifteen times* more frequently in women than men. The second most common thyroid disease (Hashimoto's thyroiditis, which causes an underactive thyroid gland) occurs five times more frequently in women. Thyroid nodules (lumps) and thyroid cancer are also much more common in women than men.

Thyroid disease can aggravate all kinds of health conditions that typically plague women, ranging from gynecological problems, eating disorders, depression (particularly postpartum depression), heart disease, and osteoporosis. Because thyroid disorders can affect one's appearance, women may suffer from body image problems or low self-esteem as a result of a change in appearance.

Why are women more susceptible to thyroid disorders? One reason has to do with estrogen. It is believed that estrogen makes women more sensitive to thyroid hormone, which means that a thyroid disorder can wreak havoc on a woman's reproductive system at all stages of her life. For example, animal studies show that estrogen can aggravate an inflamed thyroid (called thyroiditis, discussed in chapter 2), while testosterone actually improves thyroiditis, which may explain why thyroid disease is often considered more of a "woman's disease." There is also evidence that changing levels of prolactin may influence thyroid hormone, discussed more in chapter 4.

Women are also more susceptible to autoimmune diseases, which means that the body attacks its own tissue. Lupus, multiple sclerosis, and rheumatoid arthritis are all examples of autoimmune diseases that strike women almost exclusively. Two of the most common thyroid disorders—Graves' disease and Hashimoto's disease—are also auto-immune. Stress as well as a natural immune-deficiency that occurs during pregnancy (to avoid "rejection" of the fetus) are believed to be triggers of autoimmune diseases in women.

There is a separate issue with respect to thyroid disorders and women that affects a woman's emotional and physical health: validation. Since so many symptoms of thyroid disease are vague (see chapter 2) and can be masked by other women's health problems (or ignored because of the *existence* of other health problems), many women suffer from these five horrible words: "It's all in your head!" Misdiagnosed thyroid disorders can worsen existing health problems and lead to unnecessary suffering. Our current system of medicine is also frequently dismissive of women's health interests, which can lead women down a frustrating path of "doctor bouncing" in order to obtain an accurate diagnosis of a thyroid disorder (discussed in chapter 10).

This chapter is your starting point. It explains what your thyroid does, what your ovaries do, and how your unique physiology can be affected by a thyroid disorder. Symptoms of thyroid disease and the types of thyroid disorders that occur are discussed in chapter 2. If you're are suffering from a thyroid disorder, take heart: it's not all in your head—*it's all in your neck*. And it's treatable—which is something that cannot always be said about other women's health problems.

What Is a Thyroid?

The word *thyroid* was named in the 1600s and is Greek for "shield" because of its butterfly shape. Your thyroid gland is located in the lower part of your neck, in front of your windpipe (see Figure 1.1),

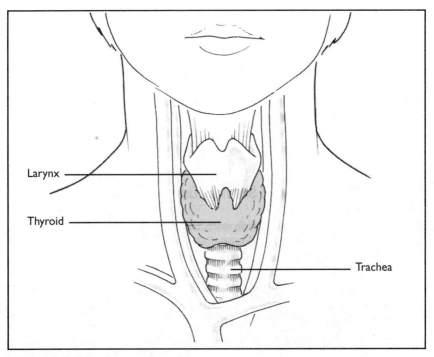

Figure 1.1 Where your thyroid lives.
Reprinted from *Nichts Gutes im Schilde Krankheiten der Schiddruse.* Copyright 1994, Georg Thieme Publishing.

and it makes two thyroid hormones—thyroxine, known as T4 (four iodine atoms) and triiodothyronine, known as T3 (three iodine atoms). Thyroid hormone (the two hormones are referred to in the singular; the word *hormone* is Greek for "stimulator") is then secreted into the circulatory system and becomes widely distributed throughout the body; it is one of the basic regulators of the function of every cell and tissue within the body, and a steady supply is crucial for good health. In essence, your thyroid affects you from head to toe—including skin and hair! (See Figure 1.2.)

If you were to break down exactly how much T4 and T3 is secreted by your thyroid, you would find that 90 percent of the thyroid output is T4 and only 10 percent is T3. Although these hormones have the same effect in your body, T3 is four times as powerful as T4 and works *eight times* as fast. It is akin to a juice in a bottle and frozen concentrate. T4 can also "turn into" T3 by shedding an iodine atom if your body requires some thyroid hormone—fast!

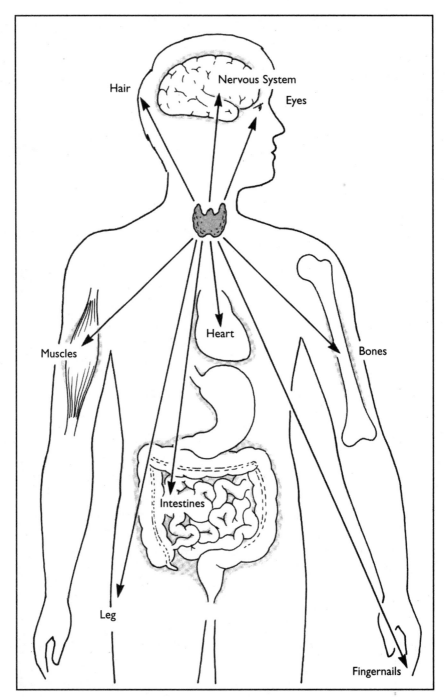

Figure 1.2 The thyroid affects the body from head to toe.

Reprinted from *Nichts Gutes im Schilde Krankheiten der Schiddruse*. Copyright 1994, Georg Thieme Publishing.

Iodine

Your thyroid gland extracts iodine from various foods, including certain vegetables, shellfish, milk products (cow udders are washed with large amounts of iodine, which winds up in your milk), and *anything* with iodized salt. Normally, we consume sufficient iodine in our daily diet.

Our thyroids are very sensitive to iodine. When the thyroid gland is not able to obtain sufficient quantities of iodine, your thyroid can enlarge, and you will develop what is called a goiter. A goiter can also develop if your thyroid gland absorbs too much iodine and produces either too little or too much thyroid hormone. Although it seems odd that both too much and too little iodine can produce the same results, the reason the goiter develops in each case is different. Usually, where too little iodine is present, a goiter is caused by increased activity of thyroid gland cells, while too much iodine can cause the thyroid gland to enlarge.

Women with goiters are well known throughout history, and as discussed in chapter 4, the thyroid naturally enlarges during pregnancy. Goiters even appear in famous paintings and portraits of women, including Rubens's *Le Chapeau de Paille,* which hangs in the National Gallery in London.

Goiter belts and iodine deficiency A goiter belt is not a fashion accessory. You may be familiar with the term *goiter belt,* which refers to regions that typically suffer from insufficient iodine. The Great Lakes region, for example, was considered a goiter belt. The term originated because inhabitants of these regions would often develop goiters from a lack of iodine. Goiter belts are located far from salt water. In regions close to salt water, iodine gets into the soil and water supply from the wind and rain off the saltwater ocean. It also gets into plants. It then travels into the milk and meat in our diet.

The introduction of iodized salt in our diet has virtually eliminated goiters resulting from iodine deficiencies in North America. But the problem of iodine deficiency is far from solved in other parts of the world. In fact, over one billion people are at risk for iodine deficiency-related thyroid disease. Three hundred million people in Asia alone suffer from goiters, while twenty million people suffer from brain damage due to iodine deficiency in pregnancy and infancy. This is very disturbing because these problems can be completely prevented by the simple addition of iodized salt or iodized oil (proposed in some regions) to the diet. Goiters from iodine deficiency are regularly found in Asia, Africa, South America, and especially in mountainous regions such as the Himalayas and the Andes.

The first International Goiter Congress was held in 1929 in Berne after Switzerland and the U.S. introduced iodized salt. Many countries soon followed suit, and iodine deficiency has disappeared in most parts of the world. But not much happened to eliminate iodine deficiency in underdeveloped nations until 1985, when thyroid specialists established the International Council for Control of Iodine Deficiency Disorders (ICCIDD), a group of about 400 members from seventy different countries.

While in North America only about 1 in 4,000 newborns is born with hypothyroidism, in iodine-deficient areas 10 percent of all newborns are hypothyroid. Worse still, up to 70 percent of iodine-deficient populations are severely hypothyroid. As a result, iodine deficiency is now recognized as the most common cause of preventable mental defects. ICCIDD works with the World Health Organization and UNICEF to develop national programs in Africa, Asia, Latin America, and Europe with the goal of eliminating iodine deficiency in the near future. Most recently, the salt industry has joined the fight, too.

A current project under way is the European ThyroMobil Campaign, which visited both Western and Eastern Europe and The Netherlands. A van is equipped with ultrasound and urine sampling facilities, and the company that runs the van has developed a urine test for iodine deficiency that delivers results in ten minutes, thus determining on-the-spot whether the person tested is iodine deficient. As of this writing, the ThyroMobil van will visit Southeast Asia.

The Role of Calcitonin

Your thyroid gland rents space to nonthyroid cells called C cells, which make the hormone calcitonin. This hormone helps to regulate calcium, and hence prevent osteoporosis. It is also used to treat

Paget's disease, a bone disease that affects mostly men. Yet, to your *bones,* calcitonin can be likened to a "tonsil"; it serves a useful purpose. But when the hormone is not manufactured due to the absence of a thyroid gland (if it's removed or ablated by radioactive iodine), you won't really notice any effects, just as you don't "miss" your tonsils. Calcium levels are really controlled by the parathyroid glands, discussed later, and are much more dependent on the hormone estrogen, which helps with calcium absorption, diet, and exercise, which build bone mass.

Calcitonin is only important in regard to the thyroid if you are discussing screening for a rare type of thyroid cancer called medullary thyroid cancer (see chapter 9). When this kind of thyroid cancer develops, your thyroid overproduces calcitonin, which is the telltale marker for this type of cancer. Once the thyroid is removed due to medullary thyroid cancer, continued calcitonin secretions are a sign that not enough thyroid tissue was removed.

The Role of Thyroglobulin

Although this sounds like a Halloween candy, thyroglobulin is a specific protein made only by your thyroid cells and used mostly by the thyroid gland itself to make thyroid hormone. Like calcitonin, this substance isn't all that important to your body once your thyroid is gone; you won't miss it. The only role thyroglobulin plays after your thyroid problem is treated is in screening for thyroid cancer *recurrence.* You see, when your thyroid gland is removed due to any type of thyroid cancer (see chapter 9), this protein shouldn't be manufactured anymore. But when thyroglobulin shows up on a blood test, it is a sign that some thyroid tissue was left that is now "active" and, hence, potentially cancerous. For hyperthyroid or hypothyroid patients, however, screening for thyroglobulin is useless.

Overactive and Underactive

Your thyroid gland is particularly sensitive to the law of supply and demand. Like a domestic manufacturer, it isn't licensed to *export* anything at all and is forced to use everything it produces, suffering the consequences of either overproduction or underproduction. If, for example, your thyroid gland manufactures too much thyroid hormone, your body will speed up. Your heart rate will increase or race, you might feel hot all the time, have diarrhea, lose weight, or feel dizzy or shaky. In a sense, the thyroid *eats the costs* at your body's expense. This is known as hyperthyroidism ("hyper" means too much) and is explained more thoroughly in chapter 2.

If your thyroid manufactures too little, your body suffers immediate losses. Most bodily functions slow right down. You will have an unusually slow pulse, feel very tired, and have no energy. You might be constipated, get a little puffy, feel cold all the time, and your skin might get very dry. This is known as hypothyroidism ("hypo" means too little), which is also explained in detail in chapter 2.

The Pituitary Gland

Your thyroid is under a lot of pressure to meet precise demand for a product it monopolizes. That's where your pituitary gland comes in. Like a government, it controls and regulates all bodily functions and secretions (see Table 1.1). The pituitary gland (often referred to as the master gland) is situated at the base of the skull and is, without question, the most influential gland in your body. Your thyroid gland reports directly to it. (So do your ovaries—which I will discuss later.)

The pituitary gland regularly monitors T4 and T3 stock in your body's blood levels. When stock is low, it sends a message to your thyroid gland—in the form of a stimulating hormone called TSH (thyroid stimulating hormone)—and orders it to produce more. The pituitary gland will secrete only increased amounts of TSH when T4 and/or T3 levels are low.

Problems at the helm When hormone levels are adequate, TSH production is quite small; when hormone levels are too high, the pituitary gland stops all TSH secretion. This should alert the thyroid to stop production. But it doesn't always work, particularly when the thyroid gland is infiltrated or under attack.

This situation occurs, for instance, with a multinodular goiter, meaning a bumpy or lumpy, enlarged thyroid gland. What happens here is that, for some unknown reason, a lump or nodule forms on

Table 1.1 Your Hormones in One Place

The Gland(s)	Hormones It Makes	What Hormones Do
Thyroid gland	thyroxine and triiodothyronine (T4 and T3)	control the heart and metabolic rate
	calcitonin	regulates calcium blood levels
Parathyroid gland	parathyroid hormone (PTH)	regulates calcium and phosphorus phosphorus
Adrenal glands	stress hormones—adrenaline/ noradrenaline	regulate heart rate and blood pressure
	steroid hormones—e.g., hydrocortisone	convert carbohydrate into energy
	sex hormones—estrogen/progesterone*	control sexual development
Ovaries**	sex hormones—estrogen and progesterone	control menstrual cycle
Pancreas	insulin	maintains blood sugar levels
	glucagon	stimulates the liver to produce glucose
Pituitary gland	growth hormone	controls growth and aging
	prolactin	controls milk production
	antidiuretic hormone (ADH), oxytocin	regulates and controls urine production, controls uterine contractions, childbirth, and breast-feeding
	thyroid stimulating hormone (TSH)	controls thyroid hormone (T4, T3)

* In men, the sex hormone is testosterone.

** In men, the testicles produce sperm.

Source: Adapted by permission from Patsy Westcott, *Thyroid Problems: A Practical Guide to Symptoms and Treatment* (London: Thorsons/HarperCollins, 1995), 13.

your thyroid gland and mimicks the gland in every conceivable way. These nodules are wanna-be thyroid glands. They watch the thyroid gland in action, and in time learn to make T3 and T4 as well. They are completely unaware of the pituitary gland, which has no knowledge that these nodules exist. The pituitary gland stops the TSH secretion, which alerts the thyroid gland to slow down production. And it does. But T3 and T4 are still produced in uncontrolled quantities from the copycat nodes. So the system breaks down, and *you* wind up hyperthyroid.

This same scenario can take place if you suffer from Graves' disease, which is an autoimmune or self-attacking disease, explained more thoroughly in chapter 8. With Graves' disease, the body attacks its very own thyroid gland. Something goes haywire in the immune system, and the thyroid gland is suddenly seen as an enemy. So an armed antibody is produced, called thyroid stimulating antibody (TSA). TSA is then sent on a special search-and-destroy mission and launches a surprise attack on your poor thyroid gland, which is only doing its job. The result is a communication breakdown between the thyroid gland and pituitary gland. Confused and disoriented, the thyroid gland makes thyroid hormone like it's going out of style. The pituitary gland again stops TSH secretion, thinking the command to "Slow Down" will be followed by the thyroid gland. But the thyroid gland's factory has been bombed by attacking forces, and it doesn't understand. Once again, *you* wind up hyperthyroid.

So, like any check-and-balance system, there is always a hole. When your thyroid is out of control, there is no way that your body can manage the situation without outside intervention. If there was, all it would have to do is excrete all excess thyroid hormone. Unfortunately, it's not that easy. As a result, overproduction or underproduction of thyroid hormone can cause both structural and functional damage.

Functional Versus Structural Thyroid Disorders

Graves' disease is a good example of a thyroid disorder from a *functional* perspective. In the early stages of Graves' disease, the thyroid might enlarge only slightly, and would perhaps not be felt by your doctor. To the doctor, your thyroid appears normal in size and shape but scores low in the performance category—overproducing thyroid hormone and causing your body to overwork itself. Performance in this case is measured by a blood test.

A goiter is an example of a *structural* disorder. (Goiters can be caused by Graves' disease or other conditions resulting in underproduction or overproduction of thyroid hormone.) In this case, your thyroid would grow noticeably larger in appearance, something your doctor could verify definitively by simply feeling your neck. If the goiter is a by-product of an overactive thyroid, for example, a blood test may determine hyperthyroidism *before* the goiter grows too large. But many times an overactive thyroid gland isn't diagnosed by your doctor until the enlargement is so pronounced that the doctor can't miss it.

Nodules Your thyroid gland is also vulnerable to a hostile takeover. For reasons usually unknown (in some cases, exposure to radiation is a cause, discussed in chapter 9), the tissue and cells in the thyroid gland mutate and start to reproduce in the form of lumps. These lumps or nodules, referred to as "cold," are primitive cells that lack the intelligence to produce thyroid hormone. So they mindlessly reproduce and mutate without any purpose or direction. Nodules are discussed in detail in chapter 9.

When these cold nodules develop, it is not your thyroid gland that is in immediate danger, but the rest of your body. When these nodules appear, their *rate of reproduction* can increase and spread throughout your body. This is known as thyroid cancer, which is explained in great detail in chapter 9. Ironically, a person with thyroid cancer may have perfect thyroid function, however. Usually when thyroid cancer is detected, surgical removal of your thyroid gland is performed to prevent the spread of primitive cells. Many thyroid cancers, however, are extremely slow-growing and may not spread elsewhere for several years.

The Parathyroid Glands

Everyone has at least four parathyroid glands that control the blood calcium level, or calcium balance. (Some people have more than four.) Your parathyroid glands stimulate the release of calcium from the bone to raise blood calcium levels. They also help your body convert vitamin D into calcium.

These glands are located on the back of each lobe of your thyroid gland. The easiest way to grasp exactly where they are located is to imagine the capital letter "H." At each tip of the "H," imagine a circle. If the "H" is your thyroid gland, the circles at each tip are your parathyroid glands.

Parathyroid glands usually come into play only when you undergo *surgical* treatment for a thyroid condition. Surgery is most commonly required when thyroid cancer is diagnosed, or a goiter—resulting from hyperthyroidism—has grown out of control.

Because the glands are so close in proximity to the thyroid gland, surgical complications could be serious. Essentially, if a surgeon is performing a thyroidectomy (removal of the thyroid gland) or simply removing benign or malignant growths on or around the thyroid gland, he must be careful not to touch or disrupt the parathyroid glands. As long as there is one good functioning parathyroid gland, there is no problem. However, these small glands are susceptible to either temporary or permanent damage during thyroid surgery.

If the parathyroid glands were to become accidentally removed or damaged from thyroid surgery, your blood calcium levels would drop. This could cause muscle spasms and contractions, seizures or convulsions, and cataracts. If the damage was temporary, you would need to take calcium intravenously and orally. If the damage was permanent, you would need to take calcium supplements as well as vitamin D for the rest of your life and have your calcium levels tested frequently. Vitamin D helps your body absorb calcium. You may be low on calcium for other reasons, too. Diuretics can cause you to lose calcium in your urine; kidney problems can affect calcium levels, and certain medications can affect calcium levels. Diet, of course, is also key: when you are not eating enough calcium-rich foods, your calcium levels can drop.

Sometimes, however, tumors can develop on the parathyroid gland itself. These tumors are usually located behind the thyroid gland and do not affect it. When this happens, surgical removal of the parathyroid gland tumor is done. Depending on whether the growths are benign (noncancerous) or malignant (cancerous—which is rare), removal of one or more of the parathyroid glands is sometimes necessary. Tumors of the parathyroid are rare and statistically occur in patients who received some form of radiation to their neck during childhood. (See chapter 9 for more details.)

Tracing Thyroid Disease in Your Family

Sometimes truth really is stranger than fiction. For example, dyslexia, prematurely gray hair, hair loss, left-handedness, and vitiligo, a skin condition that results in patches of pigmentation loss (this is the condition that Michael Jackson attributes to his "bleached skin" appearance) are statistically linked to thyroid disorders. Although these conditions are physically harmless, the presence of these inherited traits can point to long family histories of thyroid disease. In these times of rising health-care costs, being aware of your family's medical history can often save hundreds, if not thousands, of dollars in diagnostic tests, treatment, and prescriptions.

Tracing thyroid disease in the family is also important if you are either planning a family or already have children. If you are pregnant, trying to get pregnant, or *unable* to get pregnant, it is important that your doctor be aware of your family's thyroid history. If you are prone to thyroid disorders, you are consequently more vulnerable to them when you are pregnant. And as discusssed further on, *sometimes* an infertility problem is linked to a thyroid disorder. (Pregnancy and thyroid are covered in detail in chapter 4.)

If you already have children and you know your family has a history of thyroid disorders, you can alert them to that fact when they are older (particularly daughters, since thyroid disorders occur more frequently in women) and encourage regular testing of thyroid levels in their late teens and adulthood. You can also alert your children's doctors to your family's thyroid history. Again, the point is to avoid unnecessary health costs that can arise through misdiagnosis of either specific thyroid disorders or related disorders.

Statistically, dyslexia occurs more frequently in families where someone has been diagnosed with hypothyroidism, hyperthyroidism, or Hashimoto's disease (see chapter 8) than in families with a history of normal thyroid function. It's important to note, though, that the dyslexia itself is not caused by a thyroid problem. Usually thyroid disorders strike the females in a family, while dyslexia strikes the males.

Dyslexia is a *correctable* learning disability characterized by a number of things: delays in physical or speech development, poor spelling or handwriting, stuttering, right-left confusion, and reversal of numbers or letters. Although dyslexic children may have difficulty reading, and perform poorly in the academic arena, they are usually very bright and often gifted in athletics, art, and music. Dyslexic children or adults are often left-handed or ambidextrous.

If there are children in your family who show signs of dyslexia, and if your family has a history of thyroid problems, ask your child's school to suggest counselors who specialize in learning disabilities. If you come from a family with a history of thyroid disorders, experienced similar difficulties as a child, and still confuse right and left or reverse letters, you may well be an undiagnosed dyslexic. Dyslexia is not a physically unhealthy condition in any way and is "treatable" given the appropriate tutoring.

Turning gray prematurely (that is, before thirty) is a seemingly trivial family trait. It is a statistical fact, however, that premature gray occurs far more frequently in people with thyroid disorders than in people with normal thyroid function. Therefore, by tracing the genetic pattern of premature gray hair in your family, you can also trace inherited thyroid disease. Patchy hair loss is another clue that thyroid disease may run in the family.

Here is how it works: if, for example, you, your mother, grandmother, and great-grandmother all turned gray by age twenty-five, you might suspect that thyroid disease probably runs in the family. You could then alert your doctor and request that your thyroid levels are checked regularly. That way, if you did develop a thyroid problem, you would avoid the possibility of a misdiagnosis or late diagnosis.

One 1992 study found that 70 percent of Graves' disease patients surveyed were found to be either left-handed or ambidextrous. So if there are several left-handed or ambidextrous people in your family, this may be a huge clue that Graves' disease will loom large.

As for vitiligo, it is also a harmless condition characterized by patches of pigmentation loss (either white or pinkish patches) on the hands, arms, neck, and face. If this condition runs in your family, alert your doctor that you are susceptible to thyroid problems. There are not many effective treatments for vitiligo, but there are some dermatological creams that may slow pigment loss. Anyone with vitiligo should be under the care of a dermatologist. If no creams or medication seem to help the condition, there are hypoallergenic makeup bases that can be used to even out the skin tone and mask the condition.

Other ways to trace a tendency toward thyroid disease is to track how many *other* forms of autoimmune diseases exist in your family. Apparently people with other autoimmune diseases, such as lupus, rheumatoid arthritis, and diabetes (these are discussed in chapter 8), are up to ten times more likely to develop autoimmune thyroid disease. Autoimmune disease also affects women at least five times more often than men, while many autoimmune diseases commonly occur in families.

Thyroid and Your Menstrual Cycle

It has probably been a while since you were in gym class. So this section functions as a bit of a refresher course. To understand how your thyroid gland uniquely affects a woman's body, it is important to first review how the female hormones work (see Table 1.1 on page 9). Low levels of sex hormones are produced continuously during a woman's reproductive years. But it is the continuous *fluctuation* of your hormones that establishes the menstrual cycles, which can become affected when your thyroid gland is either over- or underactive.

The main organs involved in the menstrual cycle are the hypothalamus (a part of the brain), the pituitary gland, and the ovaries. The hypothalamus is like an omniscient figure, watching over the cycle and controlling the symphony of hormones from above. It tells the pituitary gland to start the hormonal process, which signals the ovaries to "do their thing." The hypothalamus is sensitive to the fluctuating levels of hormones produced by the ovaries. When the level of estrogen drops below a certain level, the hypothalamus turns on gonadotropin releasing hormone (GnRH). This stimulates the pituitary gland to release FSH, follicle stimulating hormone. FSH triggers the growth of ten to twenty ovarian follicles, but only one of them will mature fully; the others will start to degenerate some time before ovulation. As the follicles grow they secrete estrogen in increasing amounts. The estrogen affects the lining of the uterus, signaling it to grow or proliferate (proliferatory phase). When the egg approaches maturity inside the mature follicle, the follicle secretes a burst of progesterone in addition to the estrogen. This progesterone-estrogen "combo" triggers the hypothalamus to secrete more GnRH, which signals the pituitary gland to secrete FSH and LH (luteinizing hormone) simultaneously. The FSH-LH levels peak and signal the follicle to release the egg. (This is ovulation.)

To simplify this process, think of it as a thunderstorm. The lightning that precedes the storm is the hypothalamus sending out GnRH. The thunder that follows is the pituitary gland, answering with FSH. Then the rain starts—lightly at first. The ovaries are the rain, which are beginning to grow follicles and trickle estrogen and progesterone into the bloodstream. This light rain goes on for a few minutes until, suddenly, *two* bright bursts of lightning ignite the sky: the hypothalamus again with GnRH. Then, BANG, BANG. The pituitary gland answers the lightning by sending out FSH and LH simultaneously. Then the intensity of the rain increases and it starts *pouring:* the follicles burst and estrogen and progesterone pour out into the bloodstream, which is when you ovulate. Slowly the rain dies down as hormonal levels taper off until the storm stops. It is at this point that you menstruate.

Under the influence of LH, the follicle changes its function and is now called a corpus luteum, secreting decreasing amounts of estrogen and increasing amounts of progesterone. The progesterone influences the estrogen-primed uterine lining to secrete fluids that nourish the egg (the secretory phase). Immediately after ovulation, FSH returns to normal, or base levels, and LH decreases gradually, as the progesterone increases. If the egg is fertilized, the corpus luteum continues to secrete estrogen and progesterone to maintain the pregnancy. In this case, the corpus luteum is stimulated by human chorionic gonadotropin (HCG), a hormone secreted by the developing placenta. If the egg is not fertilized, the corpus luteum degenerates until it becomes nonfunctioning, at this point called a corpus albicans. As degeneration progresses the progesterone levels decrease. The decreased progesterone fails to maintain the uterine lining, which causes it to shed. Then the whole process starts again.

Menstrual cycles range anywhere from twenty to forty days, and the bleeding lasts anywhere from two to eight days (four to six days being the average). It is important to count *the first day of bleeding as day one of your cycle.*

Periods and Your Thyroid

The menstrual cycle is an important element in detecting a thyroid problem. When you're moderately hypothyroid, periods are heavier and longer, while cycles are often shorter. When hypothyroidism is in a more severe stage, you may experience amenorrhea, a lack of menstruation.

Consequently, there also may be problems with ovulation and conception resulting from either the hypothyroidism itself or associated hormonal changes. For example, in some women with severe hypothyroidism, their pituitary gland produces increased amounts of a hormone known as prolactin. Increased prolactin secretions can block estrogen production and essentially "turn off" normal menstrual cycles.

When you're hyperthyroid, periods are irregular (usually the cycles are longer, that is, the length between periods), scanty, and shorter. Hyperthyroid women can also experience amenorrhea and generally have a very difficult time getting pregnant. In fact, infertility is a common problem for hyperthyroid women.

Younger girls are also affected by hyper- or hypothyroidism. If they develop a thyroid condition during puberty, for example, they may have delayed menstrual function. If you have a daughter who seems to be in this situation or are in your teens yourself and have not yet experienced your period, request a thyroid function test. A teenager who is hypothyroid, for example, may look like a ten-year-old at seventeen. Once the thyroid problem is resolved, however, she will begin her sexual development normally.

By the same token, if you are currently having problems getting pregnant or are experiencing problems with your menstrual flow, it is a good idea to get your thyroid checked first before you undergo more extreme tests. Once either the hypo- or hyperthyroidism has been treated, menstrual flows and fertility will return to normal.

Many of you reading this may also be approaching menopause

and may be experiencing changes in your cycles as a result of your "station in life," rather than a thyroid disorder. What you may wish to do is ask your doctor to test your levels of follicle stimulating hormone (FSH) to see if they are high—an indication that you are approaching menopause. This will help sort out whether your cycle changes are related to your thyroid or your age. In many cases, it is, unfortunately, related to both.

Changes to your flow or cycle length can also be caused by stress, infections, and of course, early pregnancy (a clue that you are pregnant).

PMS and Thyroid Disorders

For the purposes of this book, the term *PMS* stands for premenstrual symptoms or signs, rather than premenstrual *syndrome*. When you are suffering from either hypo- or hyperthyroidism, PMS can be aggravated, thus worsening your symptoms. On the flip side, your PMS can mask your thyroid disorder, and symptoms of thyroid disease can be deemed to be PMS-related, when in fact they are not. So the first order of business is to review all of the symptoms that fall into the category of "PMS." Then, you can cross-reference PMS symptoms with thyroid symptoms on page 19. In many cases, there are identical symptoms!

Ninety percent of women who menstruate experience premenstrual signs of some sort. Of this group, half will experience the more traditional premenstrual signs such as breast tenderness, bloating, food cravings, irritability, and mood swings. For many women, these signs are often perceived as a sign that their bodies are "in tune" or "on schedule" and that all is well. In other words, these signs are natural markers of a healthy menstrual cycle.

Out of the remaining 45 percent of women who experience premenstrual signs, 35 to 40 percent experience the same signs of the first group but in a more severe form. In other words, they have *extremely* tender breasts, so sensitive that they hurt if someone just lightly touches them; severe bloating, to the extent that they gain about five pounds before their periods; instead of just food cravings, they may suddenly find that they have voracious appetites; instead of

PMS or Thyroid?

The following symptoms (listed alphabetically) can be linked to PMS and/or a thyroid condition.

- anger
- anxiety
- changes in sex drive (either more or less)
- chills, shakiness, and dizziness
- clumsiness and poor coordination
- confusion (extremely rare in PMS)
- constipation or diarrhea
- decreased concentration
- depression (see chapter 3)
- emotional overresponsiveness
- eye problems (see chapter 6)
- fatigue (see chapters 2 and 3)
- forgetfulness
- heart pounding (see chapter 2)
- hoarseness (swelling from an enlarged thyroid can cause hoarseness)
- increased appetite and weight gain
- insomnia
- irritability
- joint and muscle pain (see chapter 3)
- loss of control
- melancholy
- menopausal-like hot flashes (if you are hyperthyroid, you may feel hot all the time)
- physical or verbal aggression toward others
- rage
- restlessness
- sudden mood swings
- sugar and salt cravings (if you are hypothyroid, you may crave one or the other for energy)

just being irritable, they may find that they become impossible to be around, and so on. Believe it or not, even these more severe signs are considered to be very normal experiences.

However, the remaining 5 to 10 percent of women who experience premenstrual signs suffer from incapacitating symptoms that affect their ability to function. It is this group that suffers from what used to be known as premenstrual *syndrome,* more recently renamed premenstrual dysphoric disorder (PDD). In other words, roughly 1 in 10 women suffers from premenstrual signs that occur one to fourteen days before her period, which significantly interfere with interpersonal relationships and daily activities, and which disappear at or during her menstruation.

The physical changes This list is not exhaustive, but women report the following physical premenstrual signs:

- breast swelling and tenderness
- increased appetite and weight gain
- abdominal bloating (which may also cause weight gain)
- constipation or diarrhea
- headaches
- acne or other skin eruptions
- eye problems
- joint and muscle pain (see chapter 3)
- backache
- sugar and salt cravings
- fatigue (also see chapters 2 and 3)
- hoarseness
- heart pounding (see chapter 2)
- clumsiness and poor coordination
- nausea, menopausal-like hot flashes
- chills, shakiness, and dizziness
- changes in sex drive (either more or less)
- sensitivity to noise
- insomnia
- asthma
- seizures

Emotional changes Of course, it is the emotional premenstrual signs that cause the most problems. They include:

- irritability
- sudden mood swings
- restlessness

- melancholy
- anxiety
- emotional overresponsiveness
- anger
- rage
- loss of control
- depression (see chapter 3)
- suicidal thoughts (extremely rare)
- nightmares
- forgetfulness
- confusion (extremely rare)
- decreased concentration
- withdrawal
- unexplained crying
- inward anger
- physical or verbal aggression toward others

The best way to determine whether your symptoms are directly related to your periods is to chart them. Women suffering from PMS would see their symptoms vanish with the onset of their periods. If the symptoms seem to be chronic and are not related to your periods, then you can probably rule out PMS and investigate other causes for your symptoms, such as a thyroid condition.

Getting charted On a separate Day-timer®, write down how you *feel* every day for two or three months. The chart should begin on day one of your cycle, which is when you actually start your bleeding. Invent your own system for charting your changes. For example, you may want to separate your physical changes from your emotional changes and designate a number ranging from 1 to 10 (1 being less severe) to chart the intensity of your premenstrual signs. You should also note any unusual activities that might increase your stress levels, such as getting laid off from your job, ending a relationship, getting married, moving, changing jobs, or fighting with a friend or family member (see Figure 1.3).

If you compare the two dates in the figure, obviously there is more than just a change in numbers. The first one appears as though some thought and logic have gone into the charting; in the second

Cycle Day: 12   **Calendar Date:** January 14/00

Physical changes
   Appetite = 5 (10 means voracious)
   Cravings = 0 (10 means you have definite cravings)
   Breasts = 3 (10 means they're really tender)
   Bloat = 8 (10 means you're really bloated)
   Weight = 3 lbs.
   Backache = 0 (10 means you are back is very achy)

Emotional changes
   Mood = 4 (1 means happy; 10 means sad, depressed, etc.)
   Irritability = 6 (1 means calm; 10 means really jumpy)
   Energy = 7 (1 means low energy; 10 means high energy)
   Sex drive = 7 (1 means low sex drive; 10 means high)
   Stress = 6 (1 means low stress; 10 means high)

Special circumstances
   Got into an argument with Lee again. The usual. I feel fine. Just a
   little miffed.

Cycle Day: 15   **Calendar Date:** January 17/00

Physical changes
   Appetite = 10
   Cravings = 10—chocolate
   Breasts = 10
   Bloat = 10
   Weight = 6 lbs. (I'm a cow!)
   Backache = 10

Emotional changes
   Mood = 10!!!
   Irritability = 10! 10! 10!
   Energy = 0
   Sex drive = 0
   Stress = 10!

Special circumstances
   I hate my life!

Figure 1.3 PMS chart—later in the cycle.

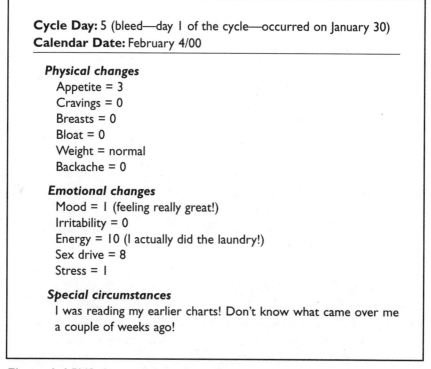

Cycle Day: 5 (bleed—day 1 of the cycle—occurred on January 30)
Calendar Date: February 4/00

Physical changes
   Appetite = 3
   Cravings = 0
   Breasts = 0
   Bloat = 0
   Weight = normal
   Backache = 0

Emotional changes
   Mood = 1 (feeling really great!)
   Irritability = 0
   Energy = 10 (I actually did the laundry!)
   Sex drive = 8
   Stress = 1

Special circumstances
   I was reading my earlier charts! Don't know what came over me
   a couple of weeks ago!

Figure 1.4 PMS chart—early in the cycle.

chart, everything—whether real or imagined—is exaggerated. Zeroes or tens. The woman was even irritated by her own chart! So it is clear that the woman of January 17th is in a significantly worse mood than the woman of January 14th. On the 14th, she was sincerely trying to be as accurate and scientific as possible; by the 17th, she was filling it out hastily, without as much care. For example, were her breasts really a "10" or were they in fact an "8.5"? The point is, it does not matter. The second chart reveals a drastic change in her attitude and feelings—a fabulous indicator of how quickly her PMS signs came and took hold of her lifestyle. Clearly, the woman of January 17th would be difficult to live and work with. Let us see how she feels after her period (see Figure 1.4).

The woman of February 4th is far happier, less stressed, and optimistic. She even has the wherewithal to observe how different she was acting just eighteen days ago, about thirteen days before her period. (Indeed, not all women experience premenstrual changes *exactly* fourteen days before their period. It can vary. Fourteen days is just an approximate number used when discussing an average twenty-eight-day cycle, which most women *don't* have.)

A word about food cravings Food cravings are a classic symptom of PMS; they can be especially problematic for women trying to manage a hypothyroid condition, which, as discussed in chapter 2, can often lead to weight gain. The food cravings are caused by an increase in progesterone at this time in your cycle, which affect all women equally—regardless of whether they have a thyroid problem. These cravings, like all PMS symptoms, will diminish after menopause. Most often these cravings point women in the direction of chocolate or sweet foods. The advice from many experts is to simply allow yourself the food you are craving in perhaps a sugar-free or fat-free format, such as fat-free chocolate pudding or "lite" chocolate desserts (see chapter 7). If you deprive yourself of the particular food you are craving, you may wind up food bingeing, which can be far more destructive and can set off a pattern of bingeing and purging, or bingeing and guilt.

Bear in mind, however, that the food you eat during this "craving period" may be responsible for an increase in weight or even a lack of energy, as quick-energy carbohydrates can often lead to a drop in blood sugar, creating lethargy and fatigue. It is also important to note that many women have less energy as a result of PMS or because of the period itself. This can interfere with daily activities or an exercise routine, which will correspondingly affect your energy levels and weight.

Thyroid and Contraception

Since the publication of my first thyroid book, *The Thyroid Sourcebook,* many women have written to me over the years asking about how thyroid disorders affect various methods of contraception. The safest methods of contraception to be on when you are struggling with a thyroid disorder are barrier methods, such as a diaphragm, condom, or cervical cap (usually a spermicide is recommended for barrier methods). Most women with a thyroid condition will do just fine on a low-dose hormonal contraceptive, such as a low-dose combination oral contraceptive or progestin-only contraceptive, which comes in the form of the "mini-pill," subdermal implants (Norplant®) or injectables (Depo Provera®). But since there are so many side effects associated with hormonal contraceptives, it is important to balance those against symptoms you may be experiencing as a result of your thyroid problem (see chapter 2 for a complete list of hyper- and hypothyroid symptoms). Bear in mind that only condoms can protect you from sexually transmitted diseases (STDs), including HIV, the virus that causes AIDS. Some researchers have found that outside sources of estrogen, such as estrogen-containing contraceptives or hormone replacement therapy, can overly stimulate the thyroid gland, which could trigger a thyroid problem or aggravate an existing problem.

Estrogen-Containing Contraceptives

With estrogen-containing oral contraceptives, your periods will be regulated and will therefore *not* be an indication of a thyroid problem if they are irregular in any way. In this case, irregular periods or changes in flow or cycle length will be related to the brand of pill you are taking and the dosage. But estrogen-containing contraceptives have side effects that can exacerbate an existing thyroid condition— or even mask it. See Tables 1.2 and 1.3 for a list of estrogen-related side effects and progesterone-related side effects. Similar to PMS, thyroid-related symptoms can merge with hormonal contraceptive-related side effects.

How oral contraceptives work Oral contraceptives (OCs) work by preventing ovulation and causing the cervical mucus to thicken, thus making it difficult for the sperm to reach the egg. With combination OCs (meaning that they contain estrogen and progesterone), the estrogen causes the uterine lining to thicken, which means that it *needs* to shed. The difference between combination OCs and the new "time release" hormonal contraceptives is that *your periods are induced on OCs*. All OCs come in a packet or case containing either a

Table 1.2 Estrogen-Related Side Effects of Oral Contraceptives

Caused by too much	Caused by too little
splotchy face	bleeding/spotting days 1–9†
chronic nasal congestion	continuous bleeding/spotting†
flu symptoms	flow decrease†
hay fever and allergic rhinitis	pelvic relaxation symptoms
urinary tract infections	vaginitis atrophic
bloating*†	
dizziness*†	
edema (water retention)*†	
headaches*	
irritability*†	
leg cramps*†	
nausea/vomiting*	
visual changes*†	
weight gain*†	
cervical changes	
breast cysts	
dysmenorrhea (painful periods)	
heavy flow and clotting†	
increase in breast size	
excessive vaginal discharge	
uterine enlargement	
uterine fibroid growth	
capillary fragility	
blood clots and related disorders	
spidery veins on the chest area	

* PMS-related symptom
† symptom can also be related to a thyroid condition

twenty-one-day supply of pills or a twenty-eight-day supply of pills. For the twenty-eight-day supply, the last week of your supply contains only sugar pills; the twenty-one-day supply requires a little more thought. You will need to remember to start your next package seven days later. Because you are off the synthetic hormones for seven days, you will get a period, known in clinical speak as "withdrawal bleeding." These periods are incredibly punctual and usually begin on exactly

Table 1.3 Progestin-Related Side Effects of Hormonal Contraceptives

Caused by too much	Caused by too little
appetite increase†	bleeding/spotting days 10–21†
depression†	delayed withdrawal bleeding
fatigue†	dysmenorrhea
hypoglycemia symptoms	heavy flow and clots†
weight gain†	bloating†
hypertension	dizziness*†
leg veins dilated	edema*†
cervicitis	headache*
flow length decrease†	irritability*†
yeast infections	leg cramps*†
acne**	nausea/vomiting*
jaundice**	visual changes*
hirsutism**	weight gain*†
libido increase**	amenorrhea†
libido decrease†	
oily skin and scalp**	
rash and pruritis**	
edema**†	

*PMS-related symptom
**due to excess androgen
†symptom can also be related to a thyroid condition

the same day, at the same time, every month. You will have less cramping and a shorter, lighter flow. You will need to take the pills at exactly the same time every day. This is to keep the hormonal levels in your body consistent.

This induced period is what makes OCs so popular. Anyone that suffers from irregular cycles, painful periods, PMS, or heavy flows will benefit from the pill—so long as they want to prevent pregnancy.

Who can be on combination OCs? If you do not smoke and are healthy, you can be on a combination OC from the time of your first period (called menarche) right up until menopause. That is because there are a number of fringe health benefits to being on an OC, known by clinicians as "noncontraceptive benefits." Because OCs prevent ovulation, they will also prevent diseases associated with the ovaries, such as ovarian cancer, ovarian cysts, and endometrial cancer. In fact, if you have no children or have no plans to get pregnant and breast-feed, staying on an OC will have the same therapeutic effects on your ovaries as pregnancy and breast-feeding because it will "give your ovaries a break." The following are considered clear, undisputed benefits of OCs:

1. OCs reduce the incidence of endometrial cancer and ovarian cancer.
2. OCs reduce the likelihood of developing fibrocystic breast condition (read on).
3. OCs reduce the likelihood of developing ovarian cysts.
4. OC users have less menstrual blood loss and more regular cycles, which reduces the chance of developing iron deficiency anemia.
5. The severity of cramps and PMS are reduced.
6. You will see an improvement in what is called "androgen-related side effects" such as acne or unwanted facial hair. (Androgen is to the male body what estrogen is to the female body; it is the sex hormone that makes his body "go.") Progestin, which is synthetic progesterone, can cause these kind of side effects, which include weight gain, acne, and unwanted facial hair. See Table 1.3 for a complete list of androgenic side effects.
7. Some brands may improve your cholesterol levels, as discussed above.

Will I get a blood clot? Women managing a thyroid condition, which can cause heart palpitations or other heart problems, should be alert to this risk because their risk of developing blood clots increases while on an OC. The rule for the general population is that if you are healthy and do not smoke, serious cardiovascular problems linked to OCs are rare in women placed on *low-dose* pills. Nevertheless, it is important to make sure that you are not *already* at risk for blood clots.

If you have a history of thrombophlebitis, pulmonary emboli, and other cardiovascular diseases, you should not be encouraged to take OCs. Your risk of blood clots forming also increases if you:

- do not exercise
- are overweight
- are over age fifty
- are hypertensive
- have high cholesterol

Unfortunately, many women with thyroid disorders who are between age forty and fifty will check off all of the risk factors above. So if you decide, despite warnings to the contrary, to opt for an oral contraceptive, you must have your cholesterol and blood pressure checked regularly.

Estrogen versus progestin side effects Many of the side effects you can experience on OCs are dose-related. In other words, if you go on a lower-dose OC, your side effects will likely disappear. In some cases, you may even require a slightly higher-dose OC—particularly if you have a history of heavy uterine bleeding. Tables 1.2 and 1.3 will help you sort out whether your side effects are caused by too high a dose of estrogen or too high a dose of progestin, the synthetic progesterone found in combination OCs. Too much progestin is what creates those "androgenic side effects" that are basically appearance-related (referred to sometimes as "nuisance side effects"): weight gain, acne, facial hair (hirsutism). The older progestins can cause a complex chemical reaction in the body that basically makes more testosterone available, which is what causes these side effects. In fact, most women who discontinue their OC will do so because of the androgenic side effects (which is understandable). The good news is that if you are experiencing androgenic side effects, it is *very* easy to fix! Simply request a low-dose, *triphasic* OC with a low-activity selective progestin which, studies show, does make a difference in reducing side effects.

The "new generation" OC When you compare the chemical recipes of today's OC brands with those of thirty years ago, it is like comparing a Commodore 64 (the very first home computer, circa 1980) with a Pentium notebook computer. In short, the OC you take now is a very different product from the OC you (or your mother) may have taken in the 1960s or 1970s.

Not only has estrogen content been reduced substantially, but so has the progestin content. The OCs of yesteryear were also all *monophasic*, meaning that the dose did not change over the course of the cycle. In other words, monophasic OCs release estrogen and progestin in constant doses. *Triphased* OCs deliver different doses of hormone over the course of the cycle. And, most recently, there are OCs with triphased estrogen *and* progestin, designed to minimize side effects. When the progestin is triphased, it delivers less hormone but is equally effective. In essence, you get more "bang for your buck." Studies comparing women on monophasic OCs and triphasic estrogen and progestin OCs show that a reduced progestin dose slightly improves your cholesterol levels, raising your HDL (high density lipids or "good cholesterol").

When your doctor prescribes an OC for you, there are three things you should ask:

1. What is the estrogen dose? Anything above 30 to 35 µg is considered high.
2. Is the OC monophasic or triphasic? (Triphasic OCs may not contain a triphased progestin.)
3. Which progestin "recipe" is in the OC? (The newer progestins, norgestimate or desogestrel, are considered to be far gentler on your body in terms of side effects. Gestodene is a third new progestin that has not yet been approved in North America but is expected to be very soon.)

There is also another wrinkle to the progestin story. The new ones are now "selective." What this means is that they are "closer" in appearance and behavior to natural progesterone, which in theory spells "less side effects."

The bottom line is that you should be able to walk out of your doctor's office with the lowest-dose OC possible to prevent pregnancy or, as I like to say: ALAP—as low as possible. In fact, ask your doctor to see all the OC samples and play a role in selecting the one you want.

Progestin-Only Contraceptives

Progestin means "synthetic progesterone" and is found in pill form; Norplant, a subdermal implant (an implant under the skin); and Depo Provera, an injectable contraceptive. Although progestin-only contraceptives share many of the same side effects as traditional combination oral contraceptives, the one unique side effect is a highly irregular menstrual cycle. Again, the irregular cycle is not related to your thyroid condition in this case. Breakthrough bleeding (meaning bleeding between periods) is the most common problem with these contraceptives.

Unreliable Methods of Contraception

If you are in the habit of using a natural method of contraception, such as observing your cervical mucus or taking your basal body temperature (both of which can be used to determine when to conceive as well), your thyroid problem may well interfere due to your menstrual cycles and ovulation patterns being unreliable and increasingly unpredictable. Until your thyroid problem is resolved, your best bet is to use a barrier method until your regular menstrual cycle resumes.

Thyroid and IUDs

If you are struggling with a thyroid disorder and are contemplating having children in the future, it is probably a good idea to stay away from IUDs, particularly since thyroid disease can affect your ovulation cycle anyway. IUDs increase your risk of pelvic inflammatory disease (PID), an infection in the upper genital tract that can cause infertility.

If you are finished having children, this may not be as much of a concern to you as to younger women. Recent studies show that the risk is highest during the first four months after insertion. Basically, the infection results because your uterus is "rejecting" the IUD, the same reason why transplant patients suffer infections. You are also at a higher risk of getting PID with IUDs if you have been exposed to a sexually transmitted disease (STD). In other words: STD + IUD = PID! Another potential risk with IUDs is an ectopic, or tubal, pregnancy. Since IUDs prevent the egg from implanting in the uterus, the egg decides to stay in the fallopian tube, which is very dangerous. Periods may also be much heavier with IUDs, and you will either experience more severe cramps or *develop* cramps. Because of this, anemia is common in IUD users. IUDs have also been linked to uterine and cervical cancers, but this area is still murky. About 15 percent of IUD users have them removed because of bleeding, spotting, hemorrhaging, or anemia.

Other complications arise when the IUD partially expels (comes out), which means lots of cramping, painful intercourse, unusual discharge, and spotting. Lost strings present another problem, making removal difficult. Full-term pregnancies have been reported with an IUD in place, but if you do get pregnant with one in, there is a 50 percent chance that you will miscarry for obvious reasons. Punctures in the uterus or cervix are another drawback that leads to pelvic infections.

The Breast Connection

There is a connection between thyroid hormone and breast development. Animal studies indicate that the thyroid hormone works with prolactin, the hormone that is key to breast development and milk production. In addition, research in many areas of breast health has linked thyroid and iodine to breasts.

Breast Cancer

At one time, there were confusing reports as to whether thyroid disease was associated with breast cancer. *It's not.* If you have a strong family history of endocrine cancers, which includes thyroid cancer (although a large percentage of thyroid cancer is caused by an external trigger, such as X-ray therapy in childhood or radioactive iodine fallout), then, statistically, you are at increased risk for developing an endocrine cancer of *some kind.* Thyroid hormone replacement pills do not cause breast cancer, nor does radioactive iodine therapy, which is based on fifty years of tracking patients who received it. While for the most part there are relatively few absolutes about the causes of breast cancer, which I discuss in detail in my most recent book, *The Breast Sourcebook,* at the present time thyroid sufferers do not appear to have a higher incidence of breast cancer than women in the general population.

Breast-feeding

The first connection thyroid has to breast-feeding is a postpartum connection: if you have just delivered a child, you may be suffering from postpartum thyroid disease, which may, in turn, be interfering with your ability to care for your infant or breast-feed properly. Breast-feeding also delays the return of your periods, which means that you cannot rely on irregular cycles to be a "clue" that your thyroid is out of whack. For pregnancy and postpartum issues, see chapter 4.

Another point about thyroid disease and breast-feeding is that you should not undergo either a radioactive iodine scan (thyroid scan) or be treated with radioactive iodine (see chapter 9). Radioactive isotopes are secreted into breast milk and can be passed on to your child.

Antithyroid drugs (see chapter 10) *can* be used, however, when you are breast-feeding, while taking thyroid hormone is also safe and will not harm your child in any way.

Fibrocystic Breast Condition (FBC)

Some of you may have been diagnosed with fibrocystic breast condition. Essentially, this is an umbrella term that refers to six separate benign breast conditions that have absolutely nothing to do with each other. At any rate, one of these conditions is known as noncyclical breast pain. This is anatomical (something inside the breast itself is causing the pain) rather than hormonal, so it does not necessarily disappear with menopause or your period, the way hormonal breast pain would. This pain is often caused by a large cyst. In fact, many women are simply prone to painful cysts. Because of this, women have come to believe that fibrocystic breast condition equals painful, lumpy breasts. This is simply not true. But women with this particular breast problem, who are told they have FBCD, may be put on an iodine treatment that has proven helpful.

Interestingly, studies show that ovaries and breasts also need iodine. Indeed, breasts have been compared to one "big thyroid gland." The breasts—like the thyroid gland—trap iodine from the blood, and it has been shown to improve fibrocystic breast condition as well as various other breast conditions. The catch is this: if you have iodine treatment for breast pain caused by cysts, you may risk a thyroid problem if you are predisposed to thyroid disease. Therefore, if you have a thyroid problem, please notify whoever is treating your breast condition prior to consenting to any treatment.

Iodine therapy appears to be widely used outside of the U.S. Many U.S. breast specialists are not aware of iodine therapy for *any* breast condition whatsoever.

ॐ

As you can see from the information in this chapter, thyroid disease can be masked by both normal gynecological symptoms associated with the menstrual cycle as well as various gynecological problems. The opposite, of course, is also true: just because you have a thyroid disorder doesn't mean there isn't another existing gynecological problem. The next chapter breaks down all the symptoms of both hyper- and hypothyroidism so that you can start to sort out what's going on.

CHAPTER 2

Signs of Trouble: It Is Not All in Your Head

What are the signs of thyroid trouble? They are symptoms of either an overactive thyroid gland, known as hyperthyroidism (when the thyroid gland makes too much thyroid hormone), or an underactive thyroid gland, known as hypothyroidism (when the thyroid gland makes too little or no thyroid hormone).

In most cases, overactive and underactive thyroid glands are *symptoms* of specific thyroid diseases; they are not the *cause* of a disorder, however. The best way to explain it is to imagine yourself with a cold; your throat is sore, your nose is stuffed, and your chest might feel congested. Here, the sore throat and congestion are cold symptoms; the cold itself is caused by a virus. Similarly, hyperthyroidism or hypothyroidism are manifestations of thyroid disease; the thyroid disorders themselves are caused by particular malfunctions outlined later on. Sometimes, to simplify explanations, doctors may choose only to tell patients that they are "hyperthyroid" or "hypothyroid," sparing them details of the actual malfunction that caused their over- or underactive symptoms. However, it is not possible to spontaneously become hyper- or hypothyroid without the existence of a particular disorder.

Often, treatment for a specific thyroid disorder results in hyper- or hypothyroidism. When this is the case, the under- or overactivity of the thyroid gland is a temporary side effect of the treatment, just the same as drowsiness can be a side effect of a particular cold medicine. This chapter explains what happens to your body when you are either hyper- or hypothyroid, and outlines possible causes of either condition. Chapter 8, which covers the role of stress and thyroid disease, also examines two of the main causes of hyper- or hypothyroidism in greater detail: Graves' disease and Hashimoto's disease. Both are autoimmune and believed to be triggered by stress. Chapter 10 outlines tests and treatments for hyper- and hypothyroidism.

Fast Women: The Hyperalphabet Soup

When you are hyperthyroid, everything speeds up. As a result, there are numerous physical symptoms that you can experience when you are hyperthyroid—so many, in fact, that I am going to discuss them *alphabetically* (see also Table 2.1 on page 42). This will hopefully give you faster access to the information you may need now! The good news is that the vast majority of these symptoms disappear once your thyroid problem is treated.

Behavioral and emotional changes You may experience a host of emotional symptoms such as irritability, restlessness, sleeplessness, anxiety, depression, and sadness. See the sections "The Emotional Effects of Hyperthyroidism" and "Hyperthyroidism and Psychiatric Misdiagnosis" for details later in this chapter.

Diarrhea Diarrhea is another sign, even if your diet is normal. Your digestion speeds up, which causes the diarrhea, and sometimes the buildup of thyroid hormone will prevent your small intestine from absorbing certain nutrients from food. If you suffered from chronic constipation prior to your thyroid problem, you may notice simple regularity without laxatives or fiber. You may even notice that you have magically lost seven to ten pounds, although you have been eating more than usual. You may also crave sweets.

Easy bruising Platelet disorders tend to be more common in people with either hyper- or hypothyroidism because your number of platelets—which help your blood to clot—are reduced. Aspirin or nonsteroidal anti-inflammatory drugs (NSAIDs), such as ibuprofen, can make the bruising worse. Your platelet function can be checked via a "bleeding time test." This disorder can exist without a thyroid problem and may simply indicate that you are more prone to develop a thyroid problem down the road. However, this does not pose any danger to your health unless very large numbers of platelets are destroyed (which is a pretty rare occurrence). A watchful eye (yours and your doctor's) remains the best approach for now.

Enlarged thyroid gland As discussed in chapter 1, an enlarged thyroid gland is called a goiter, where your thyroid will enlarge and may swell out of your neck. Here, a goiter (an overgrown thyroid gland) develops because too much thyroid hormone causes the gland to enlarge. In extreme cases, a goiter can swell to the diameter of a midsize balloon and may have been responsible for a few circus sideshow attractions in the days prior to treatment. Goiters are also caused by iodine deficiency, as well as hypothyroidism.

Eye problems If Graves' disease, an autoimmune or self-attacking disorder, is the cause of your hyperthyroidism, you may also notice changes in your eyes; they can become irritated, itchy, watery, and bulging. Sometimes double vision occurs. This is known as exophthalmos and is explained in detail in chapter 6.

Exhaustion When your body is overworked, this can lead to exhaustion, which will affect your sleep patterns, energy levels, and your general emotional well-being. See the separate section on emotions, page 41, for details.

Fingertips and fingernail changes Many hyperthyroid people notice that they have swollen fingertips to the point where they look "clubbed." This is known as achropachy or clubbing. Nail growth also increases, while the nails become soft and easy to tear off. In addition, an alarming condition known as onycholysis can occur where the fingernails become partially separated from the fingertips.

Hair changes Hair often becomes softer and finer and may not be as easy to style as it once was. In some cases you may notice hair loss and find clumps of it on your pillow, clothing, tub, or hairbrush. It may also become grayer and may not take to perms or color. In appearance, there will be a general thinning of your hair, but once your thyroid is treated, your hair should grow as it once did. To create less stress on the hair, you should avoid coloring or perms until your hair follicles are stronger. If you are self-conscious, get a wig and then take it to your hairdresser to be styled to match your normal hair. You can also contact the American Hair Loss Council at 1-800-274-8717 (also listed in the Appendix).

Heat intolerance A classic physical sign of hyperthyroidism is an intolerance to heat. Your body temperature rises, and normal temperatures feel too warm. As a result, you sweat far more than usual. The feeling is unpleasant because you feel isolated in your discomfort. Typically, someone who is hyperthyroid is constantly wondering: "Is it me or is it *really* hot in here?"

This single symptom is responsible for misdiagnosis of hyperthyroidism in women approaching menopause whose complaints of "feeling hot" are mistaken for "hot flashes," a classic menopausal symptom.

Heart palpitations One of the first signs of hyperthyroidism is a rapid, forceful heartbeat. Increased levels of thyroxine released from the thyroid gland stimulate the heart to beat faster and stronger. Initially, you will not notice an increase in your heart rate until it becomes severe.

When a heartbeat is noticeably fast, and you are conscious of it beating in your chest, you will experience what is called a palpitation. Generally, palpitations can occur from excessive exercise, sexual activity, alcohol, caffeine, or smoking. Yet, it is abnormal for a palpitation to occur when your body is inactive, not anxious, or not exposed to substances known to increase your heart rate. Yet hyperthyroid patients often experience palpitations when they are reading, sleeping, or involved in other relaxing activities. Palpitations caused by an overactive thyroid gland do not mean you have a serious heart condition, however. Once your hyperthyroidism is treated, your heart will resume its normal rate.

But untreated palpitations caused by hyperthyroidism can lead to serious heart problems and eventually cause heart failure. Normally, a hyperthyroid condition is caught in its early stages—long before any serious heart problem develops from palpitations. In fact, permanent changes in the heart are unusual in patients with normal, healthy hearts, unless hyperthyroidism is particularly severe and left untreated.

If you have normal thyroid function and take synthetic thyroid hormone when it is not prescribed (helping yourself to a friend's or relative's supply, for example), you will most likely overwork your heart and put yourself at risk unnecessarily. This is why it is dangerous to misuse synthetic thyroid hormone and why it should never be used as a weight control pill. In addition, women who use synthetic thyroid hormone as a weight control pill can drastically aggravate a weight loss program or diet they may already be on.

As many as 15 percent of all hyperthyroid people experience atrial fibrillation, a common heart rhythm abnormality. This means that your heart may pause slightly, followed by bursts of pounding, rapid heartbeats. While this may be only an occasional symptom, it is not unusual for it to be continuous until the thyroid problem is treated.

Another problem with a fast pulse rate (which may be as high as 150 beats per minute) is that the speed of the heartbeat may create high blood pressure, which can cause swollen ankles and even a collection of fluid in the chest. Shortness of breath may also develop, particularly if you are over age sixty-five. For this reason, it is not unusual for hyperthyroidism to be misdiagnosed as asthma, bronchitis, or heart disease.

Thyroid-related heart problems are treated with beta-blockers that slow the heart down (discussed later). There are also a large percentage of thyroid patients misdiagnosed as cardiac patients for obvious reasons.

Infertility Hyperthyroidism can interfere with a woman's ovulation cycle (as well as a man's sperm cycle), resulting in temporary infertility. Once the thyroid problem is treated, however, fertility is restored.

An undiagnosed thyroid problem in early pregnancy can lead to miscarriage; repeated miscarriage is often considered a form of infertility. If this is a problem for you, *please have your thyroid checked* to rule out an underlying thyroid problem.

Menstrual cycle changes Hyperthyroid women will find that their periods are lighter and scantier, and they may even skip periods. This is why thyroid problems can affect fertility—because it interferes with ovulation and regular cycles. Once the thyroid problem is treated, cycles should return to normal. See chapter 1 for more details.

Muscle weakness This is especially noticeable in the shoulders, hips, and thighs, which can make it difficult to climb stairs. Thigh muscles may in fact burn or feel soft. Shoulder weakness is noticed when you brush your hair or do upper arm movements for long periods of time. This may greatly exacerbate osteoporosis, discussed in chapter 5, as well as fibromyalgia, discussed in chapter 3. Muscle weakness is due partly to an overworked, exhausted body, and will resolve once the thyroid problem is treated.

Paralysis This is a rare symptom of Graves' disease (discussed later on), where you may experience episodes of paralysis following exercise or after eating a lot of starches and sugars. This particularly affects people of Asian descent, but once the thyroid problem is brought under control, the paralysis will resolve.

Sexual dysfunction Women can experience a decreased libido that can be aggravated by estrogen-loss symptoms at menopause. Sexual desire should be restored once you are treated. See chapter 5 for more details.

Skin changes Your skin may develop a fine, silky texture, and you may also notice patches of either pigmentation loss or "tan." People with Graves' disease also may notice thick or swollen skin over their shin bones. Also see "Hives" under the "Hypoalphabet" (on page 49).

You may also be sweating more than usual, causing your skin to become soft, warm, and damp. The palms of your hands may also look flushed, and little spidery veins may pop up on your cheeks.

Some women notice unsightly patches of thick red skin over the shins and feet, and a thickening of the skin on the fingers and feet.

Tremors Trembling hands is one of the classic signs of hyperthyroidism. This symptom was dramatized in one of the first episodes of *Chicago Hope,* where an elderly surgeon, who was about to be ousted by the hospital board because of his hand tremors, was diagnosed in the nick of time by a younger surgeon who recognized the tremor as a sign of hyperthyroidism. You may notice that you have an "internal tremor"—meaning that you feel a little nervous and uneasy all the time.

Weight loss Sometimes the diarrhea, combined with heavy sweating, contributes to weight loss—in spite of a healthy appetite. Women, in particular, find weight loss an unexpected, welcome bonus to a hyperthyroid condition, but it is this single hyperthyroid trait that is responsible for a misunderstanding of thyroid and weight loss. Usually, weight loss is limited to ten to twenty pounds, and not all patients necessarily lose weight. Hyperthyroidism often causes excessive exhaustion (explained below), and some patients wind up gaining weight because they become less active. Unfortunately, some women with normal thyroid function take synthetic thyroid hormone to induce weight loss. This is a big mistake and can cause (among a host of other unpleasant side effects) heart trouble. Weight is discussed in more detail in chapter 7.

The Emotional Effects of Hyperthyroidism

Normally, cells in the body use thyroid hormone to convert oxygen and calories into energy. When the body speeds up, however, there is almost too much energy. As a result, exhaustion can set in because the

Table 2.1 Hyperthyroidism at a Glance

Nine out of ten hyperthyroid people are women. Here's a quick check-list of hyperthyroid symptoms.

What You May Notice

- anxiety and irritability
- changes in menstrual cycle, such as no periods, longer or shorter cycle
- dry, thin skin that turns red more easily
- enlarged thyroid
- eye problems or irritations
- feeling hot all the time
- hair loss
- increased appetite
- increased sex drive
- increased sweating
- insomnia
- muscle weakness
- palpitations
- staring eyes
- warm, moist palms
- weight loss

What Others May Say

- You're moody.
- You're so talkative lately!
- You seem agitated.
- Your neck looks swollen.
- Why are you staring like that? (i.e., your eyes have a "staring" look)
- You've lost weight.
- You're shaking.

What Your Doctor Should Look For

- fast pulse
- irregular heartbeat (atrial fibrilation)
- low blood pressure
- quick reflexes
- tremor

Source: Adapted from Patsy Westcott, *Thyroid Problems: A Practical Guide to Symptoms and Treatment* (London: Thorsons/HarperCollins, 1995), 45.

body simply cannot store the excess energy. This is the paradox of hyperthyroidism: on the one hand, bodily functions speed up; on the other, mental and physical energy levels are literally exhausted. Consequently, hyperthyroid patients experience a range of emotional symptoms. Nervousness, restlessness (i.e., unable to keep still; to sit quietly and calmly), anxiety, irritability, sleeplessness (i.e., not able to sustain sleep for long periods of time—waking up every hour, etc.), or insomnia (not able to fall asleep at all) are common problems. Basically, these are linked to a general fatigue caused by very real physical exhaustion. A hyperthyroid person may exhibit some, all, or none of these characteristics; it depends solely on the individual.

Most hyperthyroid patients do experience loss of sleep, however. Under normal circumstances the body slows down and regenerates itself during sleep, which is why you usually feel refreshed when you wake up. But when you are hyperthyroid, the body continues to speed up during sleep, and patients often feel *more* tired when they wake up. This is another reason why irritability, anxiety, and general restlessness persist.

It is the emotional symptoms of hyperthyroidism that historically have caused the greatest trauma for thyroid patients. Again, each hyperthyroid patient is different and experiences a different mix of hyperthyroid traits.

Hyperthyroidism and psychiatric misdiagnosis Psychiatrists see so many thyroid patients who have been referred to them as "psychiatric" patients that thyroid function tests have now become standard industry practice for most psychiatric referrals. In fact, one psychiatrist told me that thyroid patients are the most common "misreferrals" he gets.

When women experience the exhaustion of hyperthyroidism and the natural anxiety that accompanies it but do not notice or report other physical manifestations such as a fast pulse or diarrhea (which can also be attributed to anxiety), they are often misdiagnosed. Unfortunately, it is women especially who suffer from continuous and classic thyroid misdiagnosis.

One reason for this is that hyperthyroid disorders occur fifteen times more frequently in women (see chapter 1). Another reason is that hyperthyroid symptoms often imitate the symptoms of two primary psychiatric conditions known as major depression and bipolar disorder (discussed in chapter 3). Less obvious reasons have to do with the sociological roles men and women play in the medical community. Too often, the drama of thyroid misdiagnosis involves the conditioning of traditionally male and/or paternalistic doctors and dependent female patients—a scenario that has only begun to shift in the last twenty years.

Major depression presents three main groups of symptoms. The first group has to do with depressed moods, which include irritability and sadness. The second group involves a change in physical functions including poor appetite, weight loss, sleeplessness, no energy, and a lack of sex drive. The third deals with cognitive problems. This means that anxiety is prevalent and events are interpreted or perceived oddly.

Hyperthyroid symptoms unfortunately mimic manifestations in all three of these psychiatric groups. Until the mid-1970s, hyperthyroid women were indeed diagnosed as hysterical, depressed, or emotionally unbalanced. They were often referred to psychiatrists. As stress-related ailments became more prevalent in the 1980s and 1990s, hyperthyroid women are now often told they are under too much stress. Although stress-related exhaustion is a very real phenomenon today and can indeed cause anxiety, insomnia, and many other problems, hyperthyroidism is still a prevalent and very real physical condition that often is overlooked. Chapter 10 discusses ways to become more conscious as a patient so you can take maximum advantage of your doctor's diagnostic skills. That is why reporting as many symptoms as possible remains the key. Hyperthyroid symptoms run in groups and are not usually isolated. Even subtle, physical changes can be noticed once you are made aware of them.

Finally, hyperthyroidism can sometimes cause euphoric mood swings, a characteristic of a psychiatric condition known as mania, which is present in manic depression. The good news is that times are definitely changing. Currently, there's a movement in the psychiatric profession that is in favor of prescreening for thyroid problems when

Will I become hyperthyroid?

You are more likely to develop hyperthyroidism if you:

- Are between the ages of twenty and forty
- Had a baby less than six months ago
- Had a thyroid condition in the past or are being treated for hypothyroidism
- Have another autoimmune disease (e.g., Addison's disease, Type I diabetes, rheumatoid arthritis, lupus)
- Have vitiligo

patients exhibit these behaviors. This will protect thyroid patients from being given antidepressants or other inappropriate drugs. Furthermore, when a psychiatrist suspects a thyroid condition and confirms it with a blood test, he or she will always consult an endocrinologist. At this point, the patient will probably be released into the endocrinologist's care.

It is possible for people to have a thyroid condition *and* a psychiatric disorder because both are common. In these cases, the psychiatric symptoms may result after a thyroid condition has been treated, or persist despite thyroid treatment. In short, someone with a thyroid condition is not necessarily exempt from a psychiatric illness.

What Causes Hyperthyroidism?

Although there can be several reasons why a thyroid gland would become overactive, in 80 percent of cases the cause is an autoimmune disorder known as Graves' disease (discussed in chapter 8).

A toxic multinodular goiter or a benign nodule on the thyroid gland can cause hyperthyroidism as well. See chapter 9 for more information on thyroid nodules.

Hyperthyroidism also results from taking too much synthetic thyroid hormone. Synthetic thyroid hormone is prescribed either as a supplement when treating *hypo*thyroidism or is prescribed as a replacement hormone when the thyroid is either surgically removed or deadened by radioactive iodine. See chapter 10 for more details on the treatment of thyroid disorders.

Inflammation of the thyroid gland, called thyroiditis, can also cause hyperthyroidism. See page 52.

Cold Women: The Hypoalphabet Soup

When you are hypothyroid, everything slows down—including your body temperature. Feeling cold all the time is one of the more classic hypothyroid symptoms. When your body slows down, there are equal but opposite symptoms to the hyperthyroid scenario. So again, I will discuss these symptoms alphabetically so that you can find the information you need faster (see also Table 2.2 on page 51). And also again—these symptoms disappear once the thyroid problem is treated.

Cardiovascular changes Hypothyroid people will have an unusally slow pulse rate (between fifty to seventy beats per minute) and blood pressure that is either too high or too low.

More severe or prolonged hypothyroidism could raise your cholesterol levels as well, and this can aggravate coronary arteries. In severe hypothyroidism, the heart muscle fibers may weaken, which can lead to heart failure. This scenario is rare, however, and one would have to suffer from severe and obvious hypothyroid symptoms long before the heart would be at risk.

If you're past menopause, this may aggravate your risk for heart disease since estrogen loss can lead to heart disease in women. For example, it's not unusual if you are hypothyroid to notice chest pain (which may be confused with angina), or shortness of breath when you exert yourself, or notice some calf pain as well, which is caused by hardening of the arteries in the leg. Fluid may also collect, causing swollen legs and feet.

Cold intolerance You may not be able to find a comfortable temperature and may often wonder "Why it's always so *freezing* in here."

Hypothyroid people carry sweaters with them all the time to compensate for continuous sensitivity to cold. You'll feel much more comfortable in hot, muggy weather, and may not even perspire in the heat. This is because your entire metabolic rate has slowed down as your body conserves heat by diverting blood away from your skin.

Depression and psychiatric misdiagnosis Hypothyroidism is linked to psychiatric depression more frequently than hyperthyroidism. The physical symptoms associated with major depression (discussed in relation to hyperthyroidism) cause the psychiatric misdiagnosis. Sometimes, psychiatrists find that hypothyroid patients can even exhibit certain behaviors linked to psychosis, such as paranoia or aural and visual hallucinations (hearing voices, seeing things that are not there, etc.). Interestingly, roughly 15 percent of all patients suffering from depression are found to be hypothyroid. See chapter 10 for information on the effects of lithium on thyroid function.

Digestive changes and weight gain Because your system has slowed down, you'll suffer from constipation, hardening of stools, bloating (which may cause bad breath), poor appetite, and heartburn.

The heartburn results because your food is not moving through the stomach as quickly, so acid and reflux (where semidigested food comes back up the esophagus) may occur.

Because the lack of thyroid hormone slows down your metabolism, you might gain weight as well. But often—because your appetite may decrease radically—your weight will stay the same. Hypothyroid patients can experience some, or all, of these symptoms, and sometimes, if the hypothyroidism is caught early enough, patients may not be conscious of any of these symptoms until their doctor specifically asks if they have noticed a particular change in their metabolism or energy. You'll need to adjust your eating habits to compensate, which is discussed in more detail in chapter 7. The typical scenario is to gain roughly ten pounds during a period of about a year, even though you may not be eating as much. Some of the weight gain, however, is due to bloating from constipation.

Dizziness Slow circulation and low blood pressure can lead to dizziness and even fainting.

Enlarged thyroid gland Your thyroid gland often enlarges because it is inflamed—especially if you have Hashimoto's disease (discussed in chapter 8). But sometimes, the destruction of the thyroid tissue can actually cause the thyroid gland to shrink. See the "Hyperalphabet" on page 37.

Fatigue and sleepiness The most classic symptom is a distinct, lethargic tiredness or sluggishness, causing you to feel unnaturally sleepy. I refer to my own hypothyroid symptoms as "ass draggy," where you want to sleep all the time, even though you slept well over twelve hours the night before. Your doctor may also notice that you exhibit very slow reflexes. Researchers now know that when you are hypothyroid, you are unable to reach the deepest "Stage 4" level of sleep. This is the most restful kind of sleep. Lack of it will explain why you will remain tired, sleepy, and unrefreshed.

Fingernails Fingernails become brittle and develop lines and grooves to the point where applying nail polish becomes impossible.

Hair changes When you are hypothyroid, hair may become thinner, dry, and brittle, causing you to need additional hair conditioner. Hair loss may also occur to the point where balding sets in. (See "Hair loss" under the "Hyperalphabet" for more details.) You will also lose body hair such as eyebrow, leg, and arm hair, as well as pubic hair.

Hearing problems Ringing or whistling in the ear (called tinnitus) affects approximately two-thirds of the hypothyroid population, while about one-third may actually suffer from hearing loss. This is apparently due to a shortage of thyroid hormone in the nerves.

High cholesterol Hypothyroid people can easily develop high cholesterol that can lead to a host of other problems, including heart disease. This should be controlled through diet until your thyroid problem is brought under control. It's generally recommended that anyone with high cholesterol be tested for hypothyroidism.

Hives This tends to occur to thyroid patients who have either hyper- or hypothyroidism. Hives are harmless, red, itchy welts on the skin. Antihistamines usually take care of the problem.

Menstrual cycle changes Menstrual periods become much heavier and more frequent than usual, and sometimes ovaries can stop producing an egg each month. This can make conception difficult if you are trying to have a child. See chapter 1 for more details on menstrual cycle changes and infertility.

You may also notice that you will bleed longer if you cut yourself. Anemia, resulting from heavy periods, may also develop.

Milky discharge from breasts Hypothyroidism may cause you to overproduce prolactin, the hormone responsible for milk production. Too much prolactin can also block estrogen production, which will interfere with regular periods and ovulation. As a general rule, when you notice discharge coming out of your breast by itself and you are not lactating or deliberately expressing your breasts, please have it checked by a breast specialist or gynecologist (who should also perform a thorough breast exam to rule out other breast conditions). For more information consult my book, *The Breast Sourcebook.*

Muscles Common complaints from hypothyroid people are muscular aches and cramps (which may contribute to crampier periods). In fact, many people believe they are experiencing arthritic symptoms, when, in fact, this condition completely clears up once hypothyroidism is treated. But the aching can be severe enough to wake you up at night. Muscle coordination is also a problem, causing you to feel "clutzy" all the time while finding it increasingly difficult to perform simple motor tasks.

Numbness This is combined with a sensation of "pins and needles" as well as a tendency to develop *carpal tunnel syndrome,* characterized by tingling and numbness in the hands. It is caused, in this case, by compression on nerves in the wrist due to water retention and bloating. This condition also plagues pregnant women who suffer from water retention. Carpal tunnel syndrome is also a repetitive strain injury and can be aggravated by working at a computer keyboard, for example. This condition should resolve itself once your hypothyroidism is treated.

Poor memory and concentration Hypothyroidism causes a "spacy" feeling, where you may find it difficult to remember things or to concentrate at work. This is especially scary for seniors, who may feel as though dementia is settling in. In fact, one of the most common causes of so-called "senility" was undiagnosed hypothyroidism. (So before you shout "Alzheimer's," get a thyroid function test for the loved one who you suspect is "losing it.")

Skin changes Skin may feel dry and coarse to the point where it flakes like powder when you scratch it. Cracked skin will also become common on your elbows and kneecaps. Your skin will also sport a yellowish hue as the hypothyroidism worsens. The yellow color results from a buildup of carotene, a substance in our diet that is normally converted into vitamin A but slows due to hypothyroidism. Because your body is conserving heat, and diverting blood away from your skin, you will appear pale and washed out.

Other symptoms more obvious to a physician will be the presence of a condition known as myxedema, a thickening of skin and underlying tissues. Myxedema is characterized by a puffiness around the eyes and face, and can even involve the tongue, which will also swell. See the section on easy bruising as well, in the "Hyperalphabet."

Stunted growth in children The classic scenario is wondering why your twelve-year-old son still looks like he's only nine years old. So you take him to the doctor—and find out that his thyroid petered out and he has stopped growing! This will completely reverse itself once treatment with thyroid hormone begins.

Table 2.2 Hypothyroidism at a Glance

Women are five times more likely to experience hypothyroidism than men. Here's a quick checklist of symptoms.

What You May Notice
- changes in skin pigmentation
- chest pain after physical activity
- constipation
- depression
- difficulty managing hair, brittle nails
- difficulty concentrating
- extreme tiredness and slowness
- eyelids that feel sticky
- feeling cold
- headaches, problems focusing
- irregular periods or infertility
- loss of interest in sex
- muscle spasms
- shortness of breath
- slow healing, frequent infections
- tingling in hands and feet
- weakness and muscular aches and pains
- weight gain

What Others May Say
- You look pale.
- Your face is puffy.
- Your eyes are swollen.
- Your hair looks/feels coarse. Are you losing hair?
- Your voice is husky.
- You snore!
- You used to *love* doing X ot Y—why aren't you interested anymore?
- Did you *hear* what I said? (meaning that you can't hear well)

What Your Doctor Should Watch For
- delayed reflexes
- goiter (enlarged thyroid)
- milk leaking from breasts (when you are not breast-feeding)
- muscle weakness
- slowed pulse
- soft abdomen
- tingling or numbness in the hands (sign of carpal tunnel syndrone)

Source: Adapted from Patsy Westcott, Thyroid Problems: A Practical Guide to Symptoms and Treatment (London: Thorsons/HarperCollins, 1995), 35.

Voice changes If your thyroid is enlarged, it may affect your vocal cords and cause your voice to sound hoarse or husky.

The Causes of Hypothyroidism

Hypothyroidism is often caused by an autoimmune disorder known as Hashimoto's thyroiditis, which causes inflammation of the thyroid gland, identically referred to as Hashimoto's thyroiditis (see chapter 8). There are other causes of thyroiditis as well.

Ironically, the treatment for a hyperthyroid condition often causes hypothyroidism because the thyroid is often rendered inactive to treat the hyperthyroid condition. See chapter 10 for more information on the treatment of thyroid disorders.

Sometimes a baby is born with no thyroid gland. This is called congenital hypothyroidism, discussed in chapter 4. Postpartum hypothyroidism can also develop, which occurs when the thyroid gland becomes inflamed after delivery, known as postpartum thyroiditis. See chapter 4.

Finally, 25 to 50 percent of all people who have received external radiation therapy to the head and neck area for cancers such as Hodgkin's disease, for example, tend to develop hypothyroidism within five years after treatment. It is recommended that this group have an annual TSH test.

Other forms of thyroiditis Although the most common form of thyroiditis is Hashimoto's disease, there are other kinds of thyroiditis that can occur which can cause either hypothyroidism or hyperthyroidism. Depending on what kind of thyroiditis you have, a goiter and symptoms of either hyperthyroidism or hypothyroidism can develop. Other forms of thyroiditis include:

- *Subacute viral thyroiditis* (also known as de Quervain's thyroiditis). It is suspected that subacute (or, "not-so-severe") viral thyroiditis is probably caused by one or more viruses. Although there is no final proof that this condition is viral in origin, several possible viruses have been implicated that are similar to the measles or mumps viruses, and certain common cold viruses. The condition ranges from extremely mild to severe and usually runs its own course as will a normal flu virus. When the gland gets inflamed, thyroid hormones leak out of the thyroid gland—the way pus oozes out of a blister. Then, of course, your system has too much thyroid hormone in it, and you experience all the classic hyperthyroid symptoms outlined above. But sometimes damage to the thyroid gland can result in permanent hypothyroidism, which means that you will need to be on thyroid hormone replacement for the rest of your life.

- *Silent thyroiditis.* This silent form of thyroiditis is so named because it is tricky to diagnose. Silent thyroiditis runs a painless course but is otherwise similar to subacute viral thyroiditis. With this version, there are no symptoms or outward signs of inflammation but mild hyperthyroidism still occurs—for the same leakage reasons. Usually silent thyroiditis sufferers are women, and it is common in the postpartum period (discussed further in chapter 4). This is sometimes referred to as spontaneously resolving hyperthyroidism.

Side-effect hypothyroidism Sometimes hypothyroidism occurs because of a pituitary gland disorder that may interfere with the production of thyrotropin releasing hormone (TRH). This is pretty rare, however. Tumors or cysts on the pituitary gland can also interfere with thyroid hormone production.

Borderline hypothyroidism The medical term for this is *subclinical hypothyroidism*, which refers to hypothyroidism that has not progressed very far, meaning that you have no symptoms as of now. On a blood test, your T4 (i.e., thyroid hormone) readings would be very close to normal but your thyroid stimulating hormone (TSH) readings would be high. Right now, there is much discussion in clinical

The Three Faces of Eve

If you look in the mirror, you may notice the following changes in your appearance when you are *hypothyroid,* compared to a photo taken when your thyroid was functioning normally:

- *Face:* Full and puffy, with "pads" of skin around the eyelids, as well as little yellow lumps around the eyes (called xanthelasma), which is caused by cholesterol buildup.
- *Complexion:* Pale and porcelain-like, with a pink flush in the cheeks. It may also have a yellowish tint to it, due to a buildup of carotene.
- *Lips:* They may appear to be swollen and a little purple due to poor circulation. Your tongue may also be slightly enlarged.
- *Eyebrows:* You may notice that you have fewer brow hairs.
- *Expression:* Sad, lackluster.
- *Hair:* It may lose its sheen, becoming dull. Hairspray will not hold, and you may not be able to have a successful permanent.
- *Skin:* Thick, dry, and peeling with possible patches of pigmentation loss.

If you look in the mirror, you may notice the following changes in your appearance when you are *hyperthyroid,* compared to a photo taken when your thyroid was functioning normally:

- *Face:* A little gaunt due to weight loss (in most cases).
- *Eyes:* They may appear to be bulging with the lids slightly retracted. This is a sign of Graves' disease or thyroid eye disease (see chapter 6).
- *Complexion:* You may notice soft, sweaty skin that is almost silky because you are sweating more. You may also notice that it is either increasingly "tanned" or that you have patches of pigmentation loss.
- *Expression:* Staring and almost "mad" looking because of your eyes.
- *Hair:* It may become softer and finer, and you may even notice it is falling out. It may become grayer as well and not take to being colored or permed.

circles about doing routine TSH testing in certain groups of people for subclinical hypothyroidism. This would include anyone with a family history of thyroid disease, women over forty, women after childbirth, and anyone over age sixty. Because the TSH test is simple and can be added to any blood laboratory package, it presents an opportunity to "catch" hypothyroidism before symptoms develop, and hence prevent it, and all the symptoms discussed under the "Hypoalphabet" on page 46.

༄

When you examine the symptoms of hypothyroidism, in particular, fatigue and depression can lead to some real problems with misdiagnosis—in both directions. Depression can mask hypothyroidism and vice versa. Chronic fatigue syndrome may also mask hypothyroidism and vice versa. For this reason, I've devoted chapter 3 to the complex topic of how fatigue and depression relate to thyroid disease.

Fatigue, Depression, and Thyroid Disease

If you look at the list of symptoms that comprise hypothyroidism and hyperthyroidism (see chapter 2), many of them are identical to symptoms of depression; other organic diseases such as chronic fatigue syndrome, allergies, and environmental sensitivities; or just plain old exhaustion from stress and overwork. Just because you *have* thyroid disease does not mean that you cannot also be suffering from another organic illness or even a situational depression, the symptoms of which are covered below. Indeed, being ill is often the situation that *triggers* your depression. But when you are referred to a psychiatrist when all you need is thyroid hormone, or a well-earned vacation for that matter, it can be enough to . . . well, drive you crazy!

This chapter is designed for the woman who falls between the cracks and whose thyroid disorder—or depression—may be misdiagnosed. This is the woman who cannot find relief from her symptoms because nobody bothered to check her thyroid, find out if she is allergic to the carpet fibers or industrial toxins in her workplace, ask how many hours a week she works, or when the last time was that she ate a nutritious meal. In these cases, treating the organic disease or organic roots of her "depression symptoms" *is* the cure. One of the most common referrals psychiatrists get from family doctors are women who *appear* to be depressed when, in fact, they are hypothyroid. A simple blood test and a little thyroid hormone magically restore them to their vibrant, energetic selves, while the depression disappears. These are the kinds of scenarios that this chapter intends to address.

Normal Stress and Fatigue

Before you immediately blame your thyroid gland for your fatigue, it's important to understand how sick you can feel when you're suffering from just plain old fatigue and stress due to lack of sleep, overwork, and "garden variety" annoyances. The cure is obvious: Get more sleep and don't work so hard. Trite advice for such trying times! In other words, most of us cannot afford the cure if we want to keep paying the mortgage or rent.

Fatigue is one of the most common complaints doctors hear from their patients. It's no big secret that women these days are tired and stressed. Most women have multiple roles, juggling career and family pressures. If you are over age forty, chances are that you have an ailing parent that you have to care for in addition to your own family.

There is a difference between feeling normal fatigue and chronic fatigue, which is characterized by low energy, lethargy, and flu-like symptoms—also signs of hypothyroidism. This section outlines some of the factors responsible for normal fatigue that can be remedied by making lifestyle changes.

Sleep Deprivation

Women who have demanding jobs that require long hours are often sleep deprived, which can have serious health repercussions. Recent research into sleep deprivation has found that it not only depletes the immune system (it depletes you of certain cells needed to destroy viruses and cancerous cells) but that it can promote the growth of fat instead of muscle and may speed up the aging process, too.

Research also indicates that lack of sleep increases levels of the hormone *cortisol,* which is the "stress hormone." As cortisol rises, muscle-building human-growth hormone and prolactin, a breast-feeding hormone that also helps to protect the immune system, decreases. Normally, cortisol levels should decline, while human growth hormone and prolactin should increase during sleep. Cortisol declines prior to sleep because it is the body's way of preparing for sleep.

Cortisol normally increases in the morning, causing you to be more alert. Cortisol is released by the adrenal gland in response to stress and is essentially an "alert" hormone that makes you take action. This is what causes you to be alert in important meetings, "close the sale or deal," or suddenly become incredibly articulate with someone on the phone after spending five days with two toddlers without any relief. The hormone will subside in the body as the stressful event passes.

A common reason women, in particular, cut down on their sleep is to get in their "workout time" before the day begins. It's not unusual for many working women to rise at 5:00 A.M., for example, in order to get their exercise. According to sleep experts, this will both *compromise* health and increase stress. The benefits of exercise may be canceled by the detriment resulting from lack of sleep. In the U.S., a National Sleep Foundation survey revealed that 2 out of 3 people get less than the recommended eight hours of sleep per night, while a third get less than six hours of sleep.

There are two phases of sleep: rapid eye movement (REM) and nonrapid eye movement. REM sleep is when researchers believe we dream, an important component in mental health. Non-REM sleep is when we are in our deepest sleep, which is when, researchers believe, various hormones are reset and energy stores are replenished.

Right now, roughly 50 percent of people diagnosed with depression get too much REM sleep, and not enough deep sleep, which is the "replenishing" sleep.

Child-care Issues

There is a real shortage of affordable child care in this country. And that is really stressful. Not only that, if you're a mother of young children, chances are one of them has asthma, allergies, or some other chronic condition that causes you to miss work, lose sleep, or run your child back and forth to a doctor. The incidence of childhood asthma and allergies has skyrocketed; it places a working mother in difficult circumstances as she is usually the parent who cares for the sick child. Childhood asthma is often misdiagnosed as well, which can lead to high doses of expensive and unnecessary asthma medication.

We are also seeing more chronic ear infections in children and an increase in childhood cancers. Again, this places tremendous stress on working mothers.

Aggravating Factors

Caffeine I'll make this short and sweet: many studies have shown that caffeine causes anxiety, sleeplessness, and is mildly addictive. It also worsens premenstrual symptoms (see chapter 1). Experts now recommend that you consume no more than 400 to 450 mg of caffeine per day, which is equal to two 8-oz. mugs of gourmet coffee or four cups of instant coffee.

Smoking Many women smoke cigarettes to deal with stress; people who smoke every day are twice as likely to suffer from depression as people who do not smoke. Smoking will greatly aggravate thyroid eye disease as well (see chapter 6). Nicotine may also be a drug we crave to medicate our depressed moods.

Alcohol If you tend to drink wine or other alcoholic beverages to unwind after a stressful day, be aware that alcohol can interfere with sleep patterns and is also a depressant. Initially, alcohol may make you tired, and you may think it's a sleeping aid, but it can indeed wake you up later on, causing you to be wide awake at 2:00 A.M., thus preventing you from falling back to sleep. Naturally, all of this can aggravate stress and fatigue.

Women metabolize alcohol differently than men so that, even when a man and woman are the same weight, women will become intoxicated more easily. Alcohol is also tolerated by the same woman differently at different times in her cycle. She may become more easily intoxicated just before ovulation, which can aggravate premenstrual signs. Women also tend to be "secret drinkers," often drinking alone. Moderate drinking is defined by less than twelve drinks per week and is not a daily activity. Moderate drinkers do not require alcohol to cope with stress nor do they revolve their recreational activities around alcohol. If you think you are drinking more heavily, keeping a diary of your drinking will prove useful. Just being aware of your alcohol consumption patterns can often prove enough for you to change your habits.

Diet When you're stressed and fatigued you often don't eat well. By eating properly and eating a variety of foods—particularly all colors of vegetables—you'll be in better physical shape to cope.

Chemical Reactions

It is not your imagination that more people—particularly women—are suffering from a range of nondescript aches, pains, and allergies. Exposure to workplace chemicals and toxins are putting people at risk for occupational asthma and allergies, which can lead to chronic fatigue (discussed below). According to the *Journal of the American Medical Association (JAMA)*, at least ten million North Americans suffer from chronic asthma; as much as 15 percent of asthma is directly caused by occupational exposure. One of the most notorious chemicals is toluene diisocyanate (TDI), a chemical used in the plastics and oil industries. It is also found in plants that manufacture boats, recreational vehicles, and electronics.

High-rise office buildings are another source of asthma and allergies due to poor air circulation, known as "sick building syndrome." Women who work with animals (the proteins in animal skin and urine can trigger asthma); health-care workers who have reactions to natural proteins in rubber latex gloves; and women who work in food plants and inhale dust from cereal protein and flour are also at risk for asthma and allergies.

Many women notice a significant change in their energy levels and endurance as a result of chronic asthma and allergies from occupational exposure. A ten-year study by the National Institute for Occupational Safety and Health in the U.S. reveals that asthma is among the leading job-related diseases in the U.S. Canada has similar statistics.

Building supplies The following materials commonly found in workplaces have been cited as hazardous to your health and/or well-being. This does not necessarily mean that all of the following are carcinogenic, but many of the items on this list cause headaches, rashes, and asthmatic symptoms.

- Asbestos building materials
- Cleaning products and disinfectants

- Urea-formaldehyde foam insulation
- Adhesives (may contain naphthalene, phenol, ethanol, vinyl chloride, formaldehyde, acrylonitrile, and epoxy, which are toxic substances that release vapors)
- Artificial lighting (can cause headaches)
- Toners used in copy machines and printers
- Particleboard furniture and space dividers
- Permanent ink pens and markers (contain acetone, cresol, ethnol, phenol, toluene, and xylene, which are toxic)
- Polystyrene cups
- Secondhand smoke
- Synthetic office carpet (may contain acrylic, polyester, and nylon plastic fibers; formaldehyde-based finishes; and pesticides due to mothproofing for wool only)
- Typewriter correction fluid (may contain cresol, ethanol, trichloroethlyene, and naphthalene, which are all toxic chemicals)
- Ventilation systems (fodder for mold growth inside ducts, car exhaust when air intakes are placed in parking garages, bacteria from bird feces if birds nest in or around vents, asbestos fibers and fiberglass).

Multiple Chemical Sensitivity (MCS)

This term was introduced in the early 1990s to explain a wide array of health problems and symptoms that appear to be reactions to chemicals. Among the many different symptoms associated with MCS are depression and chronic fatigue, sleep disturbances, mood swings, and poor concentration. People considered at risk for MCS include those who:

- work or live in energy-sealed buildings
- are exposed to fumes from carpets, pesticides, cleaners, and airborne allergens
- are exposed to industrial chemicals such as those found in plants that process wood, metal, plastics, paints, and textiles
- in constant contact with pesticides, fungicides, and fertilizers
- live in high-pollution areas

- work in dry cleaning, hair salons, pest control, printing, and photocopying professions

Abnormal Fatigue: Chronic Fatigue Syndrome

Seventy percent of people who suffer from chronic fatigue are women under age forty-five. Many of them may be misdiagnosed as having a thyroid condition or depression. Chronic fatigue syndrome (CFS) has been around longer than you might think. In 1843, for example, a curious condition called "fibrositis" was described by doctors. It was characterized by similar symptoms now seen in *fibromyalgia* (chronic muscle and joint aches and pains) and *chronic fatigue syndrome* (symptoms of fibromyalgia, accompanied by flu-like symptoms and extreme fatigue—discussed below). The term *rheumatism*, now outdated, was frequently used as well to describe various aches and pains with no specific or identifiable origin.

In the late 1970s and early 1980s, a mysterious virus, known as Epstein-Barr virus, was being diagnosed in thousands of young, upwardly mobile professionals—at the time known as "Yuppies"—the so-called baby boom generation. People were calling this condition the "Yuppie flu," "Yuppie virus," "Yuppie syndrome," and "burnout syndrome." Many medical professionals were stumped by it, and many disregarded it as a phantom illness or psychosomatic illness. Because so many women were dismissed by their doctors as hypochondriacs, or not believed to be ill or fatigued, the physical symptoms triggered self-doubts, feelings of low self-esteem, self-loathing, and so on, which often triggered depression. But even given the most sensitive medical attention, depression seems to go hand in hand with CFS simply because the disorder leaves so many sufferers at home in bed, isolated from the active lifestyle so many CFS sufferers once had. In other words, some believe that in the case of CFS, depression is a normal response to "feeling rotten" every day of your life. It's another example of the "if you weren't depressed, you'd be crazy" adage I use in this book.

A lot of people with CFS were also misdiagnosed with various other diseases that shared some of the symptoms we now define as CFS. These diseases included mononucleosis, multiple sclerosis, HIV-related

Chronic Fatigue Syndrome or Thyroid?

The following symptoms can indicate chronic fatigue syndrome (CFS)
as well as hypo- or hyperthyroidism.

- An unexplained fatigue that is "new"*
- Poor memory or concentration*
- Sore throat (possible if you have inflammation of the thyroid
  gland)*
- Mild or low-grade fever
- Tenderness in the neck and underarm area (tenderness in
  the neck may occur with an enlarged thyroid gland)*
- Muscle pain *†
- Pain along the nerve of a joint*
- A strange and new kind of headache you have never suffered
  from before
- You sleep but wake up unrefreshed (a sign of insufficient
  amounts of non-REM sleep, as discussed on page 59)*
- You feel tired, weak, and generally unwell for a good twenty-
  four hours after you have had even moderate exercise.*

---

*signs of hypothyroidism
† signs of hyperthyroidism
*† signs of either hypo- or hyperthyroidism

---

illnesses (once called AIDS-related complex, or ARC), Lyme disease,
post-polio syndrome, and lupus. If you were diagnosed with *any* of the
above diseases, please take a look at the established symptom criteria
for CFS as outlined below. You may have been misdiagnosed—an extremely common scenario.

In the early 1980s, two physicians in Nevada, who treated a number of patients who shared this curious condition (after a nasty winter flu had hit the region), identified it as "chronic fatigue syndrome." This label is perhaps the most accurate (and the one which
has stuck).

But there are other names for CFS such as the United Kingdom
label, M.E., which stands for myalgic encephalomyelitis, as well as
post-viral fatigue syndrome. CFS is also known as chronic fatigue im-

mune deficiency syndrome (CFIDS), because it's now believed that CFS sufferers are immune suppressed, although this fact is still being debated. But for the purposes of this chapter I'll refer to the simpler label that seems to tell it like it is: chronic fatigue syndrome.

The Symptoms of CFS

The term *chronic fatigue syndrome* refers to a collection of ill-health symptoms (not just one or two), the most identifiable of which is fatigue and flu-like aches and pains.

It wasn't until 1994 that an official definition of chronic fatigue syndrome (CFS) was actually published in the Annals of Internal Medicine. The Centers for Disease Control (CDC) have since published official symptoms of CFS. Although many physicians feel the following list of symptoms is limiting and requires some expansion for accuracy, as of this writing the official defining symptoms of CFS include:

1. *An unexplained fatigue that is "new."* In other words, you've felt fine, and have only noticed in the last six months or so that you're always fatigued, no matter how much rest you get. The fatigue is also debilitating for you; you're not as productive at work, and it interferes with normal activities that may be social, personal, or academic. You've also noticed poor memory or concentration, which affects your activities and performance, too.

2. In addition to this fatigue, you have four or more of the following, which have persisted for at least six months:
   - Sore throat
   - Mild or low-grade fever
   - Tenderness in the neck and underarm area (where you have lymph nodes that may be swollen, causing tenderness)
   - Muscle pain (called myalgia)
   - Pain along the nerve of a joint without redness or swelling
   - A strange and new kind of headache you have never suffered from before

- You sleep but wake up unrefreshed (a sign of insufficient amounts of non-REM sleep, as discussed on page 59)
- You feel tired, weak, and generally unwell for a good twenty-four hours after you have had even moderate exercise. (See below.)

A word about exercise tolerance Some CFS experts feel that "poor exercise tolerance" (meaning that even modest exercise is followed by such exhaustion and malaise that you cannot tolerate it) represents perhaps the *classic* symptom of CFS. Research into CFS has uncovered that there is indeed a biological reason for this; it has to do with a deficient flow of oxygen and energy to your cells during exercise. Oxygen normally increases in our bodies with exercise; in CFS sufferers the opposite has been found: oxygen seems to decrease with exercise. This may explain a lot! Without oxygen during exercise, various "poisons" (accumulated substances we produce naturally such as lactic acid, magnesium, etc.) can build up and reduce the efficiency of our tissues and organs. Why this happens remains to be discovered; the issue of *whether* this is happening at all still needs to be confirmed and further documented, according to many other scientists.

What Your Doctor Should Rule Out

Since there are so many *other* causes of fatigue and malaise, before you are diagnosed with CFS your doctor should rule out the following:

- Hypothyroidism and hyperthyroidism
- Multiple sclerosis
- Sleep disorders (such as sleep apnea or narcolepsy)
- Side effects from any medications you are taking
- Hepatitis
- Major depression or manic depression that predates your symptoms
- Eating disorders
- Substance abuse or alcohol abuse within two years of your current symptoms
- Obesity-related fatigue and malaise. If you are very heavy, a number of CFS symptoms could be related to your size. In

this case, losing weight may help to resolve the symptoms. See chapter 7 for more information on obesity.

- Lyme disease
- Sexually transmitted diseases, including HIV or syphilis
- Fatigue related to your menstrual cycle (fatigue is often a symptom of PMS, and estrogen loss, as women approach menopause); anemia due to heavy menstrual flow is an extremely common cause of fatigue
- Pregnancy or postpartum-related fatigue
- Allergies. Delayed symptoms of an allergic reaction can be joint aches, pains, eczema, and fatigue. Foods and environmental toxins can be classic triggers.

If no cause for your symptoms is found, you may be diagnosed with a frustrating label: *idiopathic fatigue,* which means that your fatigue is of "unknown origin." This is not very helpful, and you should find out why you do not meet CFS criteria if your symptoms persist.

Fibromyalgia Versus CFS

Fibromyalgia is a soft tissue disorder that causes you to hurt all over—all the time. It appears to be a condition that is triggered and/or aggravated by stress. If you notice fatigue and more general aches and pains, this suggests CFS. If you notice *primarily* joint and muscle pains, *accompanied* by fatigue, this suggests fibromyalgia.

It is sometimes considered to be an offshoot of arthritis, and it is not unusual to be misdiagnosed with rheumatoid arthritis. Headaches, morning stiffness, and an intolerance to cold, damp weather are common complaints associated with fibromyalgia. It is also common to suffer from irritable bowel syndrome or bladder problems with this disorder.

Causes of CFS

There is no official, known cause of CFS. But there are several theories hovering around viral agents infecting the population (the book *Osler's Web* suggests this is the case, and it further suggests that there is an active government coverup of such viruses) to airborne environmental toxins and poisons that can impact the immune system.

There are CFS sufferers who have an impaired immune system, similar to what occurs with HIV infection. This suggests there *may* be some viral agent(s) at work. But there are other CFS sufferers who have an overactive immune system. This would seem to suggest that CFS may be an autoimmune condition, meaning that your immune system manufactures antibodies that attack your body's own tissues. Autoimmune diseases are triggered by stress. The pain and inflammation many CFS sufferers report is more likely due to an overactive immune system; the flu-like malaise and fatigue is more likely due to an underactive immune system. This is why CFS continues to remain a mystery to researchers. When a body is poisoned by environmental toxins, however, it's possible that different toxins can trigger different reactions by the immune system, which may explain the paradox. Gulf War Syndrome, for example, is characterized by a wide array of symptoms. Different bodies may react differently to the same toxin, too.

Stress appears to be a major trigger of CFS, as well. When we are under stress, our bodies produce the hormone *adrenaline*, which increases our heart rate, blood flow, blood pressure, and so on. Adrenaline may aggravate the inflammation and pain many CFS and fibromyalgia sufferers experience. Stress is discussed in chapter 8.

Some experts who treat CFS and fibromyalgia believe that a lack of "non-REM" sleep may be a factor in this disorder as well. They have gone on record as saying that chronic fatigue syndrome is really a sleep-related disorder. One Canadian study deliberately deprived a group of medical students of non-REM sleep over a period of several nights. Within the next few days, each of the study participants developed symptoms of CFS and/or fibromyalgia.

Treatments

Most experts agree that CFS is an environmental illness triggered by stress. Diet and lifestyle modification appear to be effective in treating CFS, as certain "trigger foods"—foods that typically trigger allergies, or fungal infections with the fungus *Candida albicans* (processed foods, foods high in sugar or yeast, etc.)—are eliminated and replaced by more nutritious vitamin-packed foods that are organic. Since so many CFS sufferers have candida, adjusting the diet is a logical first step. Candida is a parasite that normally inhabits our digestive tract. This parasite can grow and spread to other places in the body and can damage the immune system.

Often a move to a cleaner environment is useful (changing jobs or telecommuting if you believe you are being exposed to workplace toxins; moving from an urban center to a suburban or rural area).

Downshifting, a term coined to describe people who simplify their lifestyle, shedding the urban "noise and toys," often works wonders to shed stress and can often improve CFS. This may involve moving to a smaller place with a lower monthly rent or mortgage payment, leaving a job, buying that farm you've always wanted, or just blowing your retirement money and taking a long trip. (This was known in the 1960s as "dropping out.")

CFS experts and fellow sufferers caution about taking antidepressants—often the first thing a medical doctor will prescribe. Since antidepressants have many side effects that can aggravate CFS symptoms, they are reportedly not the best solution as a "first line" of treatment for CFS. The general advice is to try cleaning up your diet and lifestyle first to see if your symptoms improve. Symptoms of depression in CFS often resolve when you start to feel a little better physically and get out of the house.

There are numerous alternative therapies that are reported to work with CFS. Review my list of CFS resources at the back of this book. Many of these organizations have Websites, monthly newsletters with the "latest" treatment trends, and so on. I hesitate, as of this writing, to recommend much of what I came across in my research because it remains unsubstantiated. But like many herbs and alternative therapies, ranging from glucosamine sulfate (for arthritis) to St. John's wort, just because they're not proven in traditional scientific studies doesn't mean they don't work. Time will tell, as will word of mouth. To date, however, diet modification is the most effective treatment CFS experts recommend, along with cognitive therapy. This is a type of counseling that helps you to "shift" your thinking or focus. (See chapter 8 for more details.)

Depression or Thyroid Disease?

Roughly 15 percent of those diagnosed with depression (which now affects about 20 percent of the general population) suffer from hypothyroidism. Women suffer from depression twice as often than men. Since women suffer from thyroid disease up to ten times more often than men, one can see how depression and thyroid disease can crash into each other. Just because you have a thyroid problem, however, does not mean you are immune to depression or vice versa. But frequently, your so-called symptoms of depression are hypothyroid symptoms. See page 71 to cross-check depression symptoms against symptoms of hypothyroidism.

Women suffer from depression more frequently than men because women in their twenties and thirties are at increased risk for postpartum depression, discussed in detail in chapter 4. Social conditions for women are often more difficult than they are for men, while women tend to seek help more often than men. In later years, women tend to outlive their spouses, and depression often results due to grieving. There is also a genetic theory (criticized by many) purporting that depression may be inherited through the X chromosome; because women have two X chromosomes, and men only one, this theory suggests that it's only natural that women would suffer from depression twice as much.

Signs of Depression

Depression is clinically known as a "mood disorder." It's impossible to define what a "normal mood" is since we all have such complex personalities and exhibit different moods throughout a given week, or even on a given day. But it's not impossible to define what a "normal" mood constitutes for you. You know how you feel when you're functional: you're eating, sleeping, interacting with friends and family, being productive, active, and generally interested in the daily goings-on of life. Depression occurs when you feel you've *lost* the ability to function for a prolonged period of time, or if you're functioning at a reasonable level to the outside world when you've lost *interest* in participating in real life.

One bad day, or even a bad week (which will usually consist of some "relief time" where you can laugh at something or take pleasure in something), from time to time, is not a sign that you're depressed. Feeling that you've lost the ability to function as you normally do, all day, every day, for a period of at least two weeks, may be a sign that you're depressed.

Anhedonia: When nothing gives you pleasure One of the most telling signs of depression is a loss of interest in activities that used to excite you, enthuse you, or give you pleasure. This is known as anhedonia, derived from the word *hedonism,* (meaning the "philosophy of pleasure"); a "hedonist" is a person who indulges their every pleasure without considering (or caring about) its consequences. Anhedonia means simply "no pleasure."

Depression or Thyroid?

The following symptoms can indicate major depression as well as hypo- or hyperthyroidism:

- feelings of sadness and/or "empty mood"*
- difficulty sleeping (waking up frequently in the middle of the night)†
- loss of energy and feelings of fatigue and lethargy*
- change in appetite (usually a loss of appetite)*†
- difficulty thinking, concentrating, or making decisions (see section below)*
- loss of interest in formerly pleasurable activities, including sex*
- anxiety or panic attacks (characterized by racing heart)†
- obsessing over negative experiences or thoughts
- feeling guilty, worthless, hopeless, or helpless
- feeling restless and irritable†
- thinking about death or suicide

*represents signs of hypothyroidism
†represents signs of hyperthyroidism

Different people have different ways of expressing anhedonia. You might tell your friends, for example, that you don't "have any desire" to do X or Y; you can't "get motivated"; or X or Y just doesn't "hold your interest or attention." You may also notice that the sense of satisfaction from a job well done is simply gone, which is particularly debilitating in the workplace or in a place of learning. For example, artists (photographers, painters, writers) may find that the passion has gone out of their work.

Many of the symptoms of depression hinge on this "loss of pleasure" symptom, however. One of the reasons that weight loss is so common in depression (typically, people may notice as much as a ten-pound drop in their weight) is because food no longer gives them pleasure, or cooking no longer gives them pleasure. The sense of satisfaction we get from having a clean home or clean kitchen may also disappear. Therefore, tackling the chore of cleaning up our kitchen in order to prepare food may be too taxing, contributing to a lack of interest in food.

Of course, gaining weight is also not unusual: ten pounds in the opposite direction can occur, too. This is often due to poor nutrition as well: because we fill up on snack foods, or high-calorie, low-nutrient foods, we're not motivated to eat or prepare well-balanced meals. Weight gain may also result from a loss of interest in physical activities: exercising, sports, or a dozen other things that keep us active when we're feeling "ourselves."

A loss of interest in sex aggravates matters if we are in a sexual relationship with someone. Again, the decreased desire for sex stems from general anhedonia.

When you can't think clearly Another debilitating feature of depression is finding that you simply can't concentrate or think clearly. You feel scattered, disorganized, and unable to prioritize. This usually hits hardest in the workplace or a center of learning and can severely impair your on-the-job performance. You may miss important deadlines, important meetings, or find you can't focus when you do go to meetings. When you can't think clearly, you can be overwhelmed with feelings of helplessness or hopelessness. "I can't even perform a simple task such as X anymore" may dominate your thoughts, while you become more disillusioned with your dwindling productivity.

When you can't sleep The typical sleep pattern of a depressed person is to go to bed at the normal time, only to wake up around two in the morning, and find she can't get back to sleep. Endless hours are spent watching television to pass the time or simply tossing and turning, usually obsessing over negative experiences or thoughts. Lack of sleep affects our ability to function and leads to increased irritability, lack of energy, and fatigue. Insomnia, by itself, is not a sign of depression, but when viewing depression as a package of symptoms, the inability to fall or stay asleep can aggravate all the other symptoms. In some cases, people who are depressed will oversleep, requiring ten to twelve hours of sleep every night.

These symptoms refer to major depression, the "cold and flu" of mood disorders for psychiatrists. There are many kinds of mood disorders, however, which are covered in more detailed books on depression. Manic-depression, known as bipolar disorder, is discussed on page 75, as hyperthyroid symptoms can sometimes be confused with symptoms of mania and vice versa.

Managing Depression

When you are suffering from the symptoms of depression, the first order of business is to regain your normal functioning self again. Long-term strategies to prevent recurrence will vary, depending on the circumstances of your depression and the type of depression you're suffering from. There is no one way to manage depression because different things work for different women. Less invasive solutions involve finding someone to talk to. This translates into finding counseling or psychotherapy. Talk therapy may also work best in combination with antidepressants or herbal remedies, such as St. John's wort.

Herbal remedies In 1997, the American Psychiatric Association stated that the herb St. John's wort can be started as a "first-line" treatment for mild to moderate depression. The herb is named after St. John, the patron saint of nurses, while "wort" is simply Old English for "plant." It is essentially the "nurse's plant." St. John's wort can apparently work as well in many people as a prescription antidepressant because it relieves stress. It is also known, therefore, to relieve other stress-related problems, including gastrointestinal ailments.

St. John's wort has been used successfully for years throughout Europe, while studies show that it can do the same job as antidepressants without as many side effects.

Another natural compound shown to help alleviate depression is SAM-e (pronounced "sammy," which is short for S-adenosylmethionine, a compound made by your body's cells). Introduced in the United States in March 1999, SAM-e also helps relieve joint pain and improves liver function.

Antidepressants Antidepressants work on your brain chemistry. There are several types of prescription antidepressants known as heterocyclics, monamine oxidase inhibitors (MAOIs), and selective seritonin reuptake inhibitors (SSRIs). A subtype of SSRIs, called MSRIs, which stands for mixed seritonin reuptake inhibitors, is also popular, and includes serotonin-norephinephrine reuptake inhibitors (SNRIs). There are other kinds of antidepressants used as well.

Long-term solutions Preventing recurrence of a depressive episode involves prolonged therapy: long-term counseling and/or psychotherapy instead of short-term; long-term talk therapy in combination with medications or herbs; lifestyle changes (ranging from stress-reduction techniques to dramatic changes involving residence, jobs, and interpersonal relationships). Because long-term solutions often involve making dramatic changes in your lifestyle, which can take a long time to come to terms with, or implement, counseling is often a key component in managing depression.

Hypothyroidism and Seasonal Affective Disorder (SAD)

Symptoms of hypothyroidism have a lot in common with symptoms of seasonal affective disorder (SAD), a "blue mood" that is triggered by a decrease in sunlight related to changes in seasons. The typical person with SAD will notice that they sleep too much and eat too much (thereby gaining weight). Then they begin to "wake up" in the spring, and can even be slightly manic (known as hypomanic). (Occasionally, the reverse occurs, and depression comes on during the summer months instead; at this time, symptoms of major depression present themselves. Some of this may be related to extreme discomfort in humid, hot weather with a resulting inability to sleep, increased pollutants in the air, and all the other miseries of humid, hot, urban summers.)

SAD strikes women in their twenties and thirties and occurs with increased frequency in higher latitudes. Light at the end of the tunnel is in sight for women with SAD—literally. Sitting under bright light for extended periods is the recommended treatment, which you should discuss with your doctor.

Bipolar Disorder and Hypothyroidism

Bipolar disorder means "two moods." When you suffer from two moods, one will be high and one will be low. Bipolar disorder is the new label for an older, probably more accurate one: manic-depression, which means that the moods fluctuate between mania (incredible "highs") and depression (incredible "lows"). Although how "incredible" the high or low is can vary dramatically, which has given rise to different kinds of bipolar disorders.

For the purposes of this book, however, it's important to note the signs of mania, which can often be confused with the emotional symptoms of hyperthyroidism (see chapter 2). Studies also reveal that one-quarter to one-half of all people with bipolar disorder also suffer from a thyroid problem. Some women "recognize" themselves in the signs below, but often it is family members or friends who notice the following:

- erratic behavior, characterized by wild spending sprees, sexual "flings," and impulsive acts
- incredible bursts of energy and activity
- restlessness (constantly looking for something to do; not able to focus for a long time on one activity)
- fast talking to keep up with a "racing mind"
- acting and feeling "high" or euphoric

- extreme irritability and distractibility
- not requiring sleep (you feel there is too much to do in life and that sleep is a waste of time, even though the lack of it may lead to irritability and agitation)
- the belief in unusual or unrealistic abilities and "powers" (for example, it is not unusual for women with bipolar disorder to believe they are agents of God, or even God)
- making decisions and judgments that seem out of character or "not like her"
- increased need or desire for sex
- drug abuse (some common culprits: cocaine, alcohol, sleeping pills)
- behavior that pushes other people's buttons (aggressive or intrusive acts; acting like an agitator)
- total denial that "something's wrong" when confronted
- increasingly sensitive to sound and easily irritated by various sounds
- feeling you are extraordinary or brilliant (even though this *may* be true)
- feeling at one with nature, and having heightened senses (everything smells, tastes, sounds, feels, and looks beautiful and exquisite)
- being told you are a workaholic because you are taking on too many projects at once
- calling people all the time for no good reason, and keeping them tied up with useless conversations

❧

Thyroid disease can affect your sexual function as much as it can your emotional function (which can also affect your libido). The next chapter explains how your thyroid can interfere with baby-making, as well as life after you've had a baby. Postpartum thyroid disease is often misdiagnosed as postpartum depression, which I discuss more appropriately under pregnancy and fertility issues.

CHAPTER 4

Fertility, Pregnancy, and the Thyroid

There are two groups of women reading this chapter. The first group is concerned about *first* developing a thyroid problem during or after pregnancy, while the second group is concerned about how a diagnosis of thyroid disease prior to conception will interfere with conception or pregnancy. This chapter will address all of these concerns.

If you are in the first group, you have reason to worry about a thyroid problem because autoimmune thyroid disorders such as Graves' disease or Hashimoto's disease are most likely to strike during the first trimester of a pregnancy and within the first six months after delivery. If you are in the second group, you have less reason to worry because once your thyroid condition is brought under control, it shouldn't interfere with conception or pregnancy if you're under the care of a good doctor. That said, you should note that autoimmune disorders tend to improve anyway during a pregnancy but can worsen after delivery. So don't be surprised if you suddenly notice a flare-up of thyroid symptoms after delivery. Graves' disease, Hashimoto's thyroiditis, and postpartum thyroiditis are the most common thyroid problems that will develop during or after pregnancy.

Getting Pregnant

As discussed in chapter 1, when your thyroid gland is over- or underactive, it can interfere with your menstrual cycle and subsequently interfere with ovulation. This could make conception difficult. So the first rule when planning a pregnancy is to have your thyroid checked, especially if thyroid disease runs in your family. Your partner should also have his thyroid checked, as thyroid disease in men can interfere with sperm count and libido.

Infertility

If a thyroid problem is interfering with your menstrual cycle, it's important to remember that infertility is always temporary when it's caused by either hypo- or hyperthyroidism. Once the thyroid problem is treated, your cycles should return to normal. That said, there could be other causes for your ovulation problems. Currently, the most common reason for difficulty ovulating is age. Fertility actually begins to decline after age twenty-five and continues to decline considerably after age thirty. Ninety-seven percent of all twenty-year-old women are fertile; by age forty-five that number dwindles to 5 percent. As women age, there is also an increase in conditions such as endometriosis, when pieces of uterine lining (the endometrium) grow outside of the uterus and can block the fallopian tubes or scar the ovaries. In short, delaying childbearing is probably the most common reason why women suffer from infertility (see Table 4.1).

Casual, unprotected sexual encounters earlier in life have also led to an explosion in sexually transmitted diseases (STDs), which can damage reproductive organs (particularly in women), causing infertility in the thirties and forties. It's estimated that at least half of all infertility is 100 percent preventable through safe sex.

It's important to note that hypothyroidism is more common in women with polycystic ovary syndrome, as well as women with Turner's syndrome, a genetic disorder where the ovaries do not make eggs without female hormone supplements. For more information about infertility consult my book, *The Fertility Sourcebook*.

Having sex Conceiving may be difficult when you are hypo- or hyperthyroid because your desire for sex can be diminished. Because of the exhaustion or fatigue that sets in, you might find that you simply don't have the energy or desire for sex. This is a temporary problem that clears up when your thyroid problem is treated.

TABLE 4.1 Thyroid or Age?

Fertility declines naturally as you age. Before you blame your thyroid gland, read this:

Age	Likelihood of getting pregnant*	Likelihood of infertility
20–24	100%	3%
25–29	94%	5%
30–34	86%	8%
35–39	70%	15%
40–44	36%	32%
45–49	5%	69%
50	0%	100%

*Presumes optimum health

Source: Adapted from Masood Khatamee, M.D. "Infertility: A Preventable Epidemic?" *International Journal of Fertility* 33, no. 4, (1988): 246-51.

Other causes of infertility It's important to rule out male-factor infertility first, before you undergo an invasive workup. This is done through a simple semen analysis. Male-factor infertility is often structural, too, caused by blockages within the male reproductive tract. There is also a problem with declining sperm counts, which have been linked to environmental pollution.

In general, when infertility is caused by a male or female hormonal disorder, only a small fraction of these disorders are due to a thyroid problem.

Bad habits Eating well and cutting down on the "bad stuff" can also improve your chances for conception. For example, smoking, alcohol, and caffeine can impair fertility. Consult my book, *The Fertility Sourcebook*, for more details.

If You Have Already Been Treated for Thyroid Disease

If you are hypothyroid or are taking thyroid replacement hormone from a thyroid condition prior to pregnancy, thyroid hormone replacement (levothyroixine sodium)—the usual treatment—is fine.

Very little thyroid hormone will cross over from you to the fetus. Sometimes a change in dosage is needed because requirements for thyroid hormone can increase during pregnancy; you usually need more to compensate for a natural drain in energy. It's normal to require as much as a 40 to 50 percent increase in your dosage. In this case, doctors generally monitor the TSH level anyway and will increase your dosage as necessary.

If you've been treated for hypothyroidism and are planning to get pregnant, you should have your thyroid levels checked again while you are trying to conceive. To make sure you're taking enough thyroid replacement hormone, request both a thyroid function test (checking T3 and T4 levels) as well as a TSH test. That way, you will minimize any possible risk to yourself or your baby from hypothyroidism during pregnancy. Since you naturally feel increasingly tired when you're pregnant, fatigue caused by hypothyroidism could severely lower your energy levels.

If you're being treated for hyperthyroidism via radioactive iodine, you shouldn't plan to get pregnant for about six months. As a precaution, all doctors screen for pregnancy first before radioactive iodine is administered.

If you're taking antithyroid medications and are planning to get pregnant, you can safely become pregnant while continuing to take this medication—as long as you're under the supervision of a physician. In fact, this may protect the baby in your womb from the effects of thyroid-stimulating antibody, which crosses from you into the baby's circulation.

Being Pregnant

It was customary in ancient Egypt to tie a fine thread around the neck of a young bride; when it broke, it meant she was pregnant. It's normal for the thyroid gland to enlarge slightly during pregnancy because the fetus takes iodine away from you, while iodine is also lost through more frequent urination. The more iodine-deficient a woman is (especially if she lives in an iodine-deficient area), the more enlarged her thyroid becomes. The thyroid usually increases in volume by 30 percent between eighteen and thirty-six weeks into pregnancy. It's also believed that the gland enlarges because human chorionic gonadotropin (HCG), a hormone formed in the placenta, can mildly stimulate the thyroid gland. Researchers have found that HCG has a very similar molecular structure to TSH (thyroid stimulating hormone). (As a precaution, however, even a modestly enlarged thyroid gland or goiter should be checked.)

Normal, healthy, pregnant women often develop symptoms and signs that suggest hyperthyroidism, such as a rapid pulse or palpitations, sweating, and heat intolerance. This is because the metabolic rate increases during pregnancy. Despite this, hyperthyroidism occurs only in about one in a thousand pregnancies. Thyroid hormone levels also increase during pregnancy because of the high levels of estrogen a pregnant body secretes. This is due to an increase in a binding protein in the blood that holds thyroxine there. The amount of thyroxine available to the tissues, however, is not increased, and the increased thyroid levels would not interfere with thyroid hormone production in normal pregnant women.

Gestational Thyroid Disease
(Thyroid Disease During Pregnancy)

If hypothyroidism is suspected while you're pregnant, your doctor will give you a TSH test. Just as in nonpregnant women, your TSH levels will be increased if you're hypothyroid, and you'll be treated with thyroid hormone replacement. Sometimes, pregnancy itself can mask hypothyroid symptoms. For example, constipation, puffiness, and fatigue are all traits of pregnancy as well. If this is what's happening, your hypothyroidism is probably not that severe, but the symptoms will persist after delivery.

Hyperthyroidism during pregnancy is more complex, and when it does happen, it's due usually to Graves' disease. Diagnosis and treatment of hyperthyroidism during pregnancy presents some unique fetal and maternal considerations, however.

First, the risk of miscarriage and stillbirth is increased if hyperthyroidism goes untreated. Second, the overall risks to you and the baby increase if the disease persists or is first recognized late in pregnancy.

As in nonpregnant women, specific hyperthyroid symptoms usually indicate a problem, but here again, some of the classic symptoms such as heat intolerance or palpitations can mirror classic pregnancy traits. Usually, symptoms such as bulgy eyes or a pronounced goiter give Graves' disease away. But because radioactive iodine scans or treatment are never performed during pregnancy, hyperthyroidism—in this case—can only be confirmed through a blood test. (If, by some fluke, you are exposed to radioactive iodine during pregnancy because the pregnancy was not suspected, you may want to discuss the possibility of a therapeutic abortion with your practitioner.)

The treatment for hyperthyroidism in pregnancy is antithyroid medication. Propylthiouracil (PTU) or methimazole are most commonly used, but PTU is the one usually used during pregnancy because it does not cross the placenta as easily as methimazole. The antithyroid medication in pregnancy is used first to control the hyperthyroidism. Then, the aim is to administer the lowest dose possible to maintain the thyroid hormone levels in the "high normal" or maximum-without-risk range. These smaller doses of medication will pose minimum risk to the baby. With higher doses, the drugs cross the placenta into the baby's bloodstream and can ultimately affect the baby's thyroid. Because thyroid-stimulating antibodies also cross the placenta, they can cause fetal hyperthyroidism, which is very dangerous and may even cause fetal death. Therefore, the PTU, by suppressing the fetal thyroid, actually benefits the fetus.

Sometimes women discover they are allergic to PTU. If this happens, methimazole is used instead. When there is a problem with both drugs, sometimes a thyroidectomy during the second trimester is performed. This is rare, though. In general, surgery is avoided during pregnancy because it can trigger a miscarriage.

Many times, hyperthyroidism becomes milder as the pregnancy progresses. When this happens, antithyroid medication can be tapered off slowly as the pregnancy reaches full term, and often normal thyroid function resumes after delivery.

On the other hand, when Graves' disease is the cause of hyperthyroidism in pregnancy, the hyperthyroidism will need to be controlled throughout pregnancy to avoid either severe hyperthyroidism or complications during labor and delivery. Sometimes, beta-blockers (heart medication) such as propanalol are added to PTU, which can be continued safely during the nursing period.

A word about morning sickness If you are suffering from severe morning sickness in early pregnancy, this may be a sign of hyperthyroidism. It's believed that morning sickness can become increasingly severe because of the overproduction of thyroid hormone. See your doctor if your morning sickness is severe. Even if you do not have hyperthyroidism, severe morning sickness can lead to dehydration and should be treated.

The Risk of Miscarriage

Studies indicate a 32 percent risk of miscarriage in women with antithyroid antibodies compared to a 16 percent risk in women without them. The risk of miscarriage risk rises due to age. In the general population, 1 in 6 pregnancies ends in miscarriage with risk at its highest point during the first trimester.

Bleeding in the first trimester Bleeding during pregnancy is not normal, but it's not *unusual* either. Nor does it mean that a miscarriage is imminent. It's also important to note whether any pain accompanies your staining or bleeding. Staining or bleeding with no pain is better news than staining or bleeding and cramps. Bleeding or spotting of *any* kind during this stage should be reported immediately to avoid any risk.

The most dangerous kind of bleeding at this point is heavy bleeding. The definition of heavy bleeding means that you need to change your pads about every hour. Other danger signs to watch out for are other symptoms accompanying the bleeding such as cramps, pain in the abdomen, fever, weakness, and possible vomiting. If the blood has clumps of tissue in it, this is also a bad sign. If this is the case, save your pad. Just stick your whole pad—clumps and all—in a plastic bag and save it for the doctor to inspect. The clumps may provide important clues as to what is going on. You may also notice an unusual odor. If light bleeding or spotting continues for more than three days, this is another, less obvious danger sign.

Symptoms of miscarriage Heavy bleeding and cramping anywhere between the end of the second month to the end of the third month are classic signs that you're in the process of miscarrying. Cramps without bleeding are also a danger sign that you're miscarrying. The bleeding can be heavy enough to saturate several pads within an hour or may be "manageable" and more like a heavy period. You may also be experiencing *unbearable* cramping that renders you incapacitated. Sometimes, you can *"pass clots,"* which are dark red clumps that appear to be small pieces of raw beef liver. Sometimes, you may even pass gray or pink tissue. A miscarriage can also be occurring if you have persistent, light bleeding and more mild cramping at this stage.

When you miscarry prior to twenty weeks, it's actually called a *spontaneous abortion.* There are several kinds of spontaneous abortions:

- *Threatened abortion:* Your cervix is still closed and holding everything securely, but you're having cramps, bleeding, or staining. Your doctor will examine you and check the fetal heartbeat. You may also need an ultrasound. Then, you will be ordered to bed. In some cases, the bleeding will stop and pregnancy will continue normally. Sometimes, you might miscarry anyway because of unsalvageable problems such as severe genetic deformities.
- *Inevitable abortion:* In this case, nature has already taken its course and the process of miscarriage has started. Bleeding is heavy, cramps increase, and the cervix begins to dilate. You may wind up expelling everything while it's still intact: the fetus, amniotic sac, and placenta, accompanied by a lot of blood. This is the most traumatic kind of first trimester miscarriage.
- *Incomplete abortion:* This is when you're not naturally expelling all of the uterine's contents. Some, but not all, pregnancy tissue has been spontaneously expelled; usually what remains are fragments of the placenta. This needs to be corrected with a dilation and curettage (D&C) procedure that will clean out the uterus and help it to heal.
- *A complete abortion:* This is when all pregnancy tissue is passed spontaneously. You will *slowly* expel everything by

steadily bleeding. This will feel like a miserable period but everything will come out in time. You still may need a D&C just to clean out little bits of tissue left behind, but this usually isn't necessary. The bleeding can actually go on for days until complete.

- *Missed abortion:* This is also very traumatic. The fetus dies in the uterus but doesn't come out. You may not have symptoms indicating that anything is wrong for quite some time. This is when you just spot lightly, and may mistake it for "good bleeding." In this situation, all of your pregnancy symptoms will gradually disappear and you—obviously— won't progress at all. This condition is frequently diagnosed during a routine exam, and the fetal heartbeat can no longer be heard. Treatment depends on the duration of the pregnancy.

Finding a Solitary Thyroid Nodule During Pregnancy

If you discover a lump on your thyroid gland during pregnancy, investigation and treatment will vary depending on what stage you are in.

If you are in the first trimester, a needle biopsy will be done to determine whether the lump is benign or malignant. If it is malignant, surgery will probably be performed during the second trimester, which is considered the safest time for surgery. If a cancerous nodule is confirmed in the second trimester, surgery may still be performed if there is time. Otherwise, you might simply have to wait until you deliver. As discussed in chapter 9, thyroid cancer grows very slowly and the extra few months won't make a difference in the overall treatment scenario.

If, however, a nodule is only first discovered into the second or third trimesters, investigation and treatment can probably wait until you deliver. Then, you will be able to have a scan.

After the Baby Is Born

During pregnancy, your immune system is naturally suppressed to prevent your body from rejecting the fetus. After pregnancy, your immune system "turns on" again. But this has a "rebound" effect in that it is so alert, it is almost too powerful and can develop antibodies that attack normal tissue. This is what's known as an autoimmune disorder and may be one reason why women are more prone to auto-immune disorders after pregnancy. I liken the scenario to having a guard dog tied up for nine months (during the pregnancy) and then "let out." The dog will be more feisty and may even attack his owner.

If you first develop an autoimmune thyroid disease, such as Graves' disease or Hashimoto's disease after you deliver, you would undergo normal treatment for either disease. If you developed Graves' disease after delivery, however, you would not have to discontinue breast-feeding; the antithyroid medication, propylthiouracil, doesn't cross into your milk and is safe for lactating women.

If you had developed Graves' disease during pregnancy, the condition can get worse after delivery unless antithyroid drugs are continued.

If you were diagnosed and successfully treated for Graves' disease prior to pregnancy, you can sometimes suffer a relapse after delivery. But depending on the severity of Graves' disease after delivery, some women can opt to postpone treatment until they're finished breast-feeding.

Postpartum Thyroiditis

Postpartum thyroiditis means "inflammation of the thyroid gland after delivery" and is often the culprit behind the so-called "postpartum blues." Postpartum thyroiditis occurs in 5 to 18 percent of all postpartum women and usually lasts six to nine months before it resolves on its own.

Postpartum thyroiditis is a general label referring to silent thyroiditis (see chapter 2) occurring after delivery—causing mild hyperthyroidism or a short-lived Hashimoto's-type of thyroiditis—causing mild hypothyroidism. Until quite recently, the mild hypo- and hyperthyroid symptoms were attributed simply to symptoms of postpartum depression, those notorious "postpartum blues" thought to be caused by the dramatic hormonal changes women experience after pregnancy. But recent studies indicate that as many as 18 percent of all pregnant women experience transient (i.e., short-lived) thyroid problems and subsequent mild forms of hyperthyroidism or hypothyroidism. This statistic does not account for the many women who develop Graves' disease either during or after pregnancy.

Usually, the silent thyroiditis or short-lived Hashimoto's thyroiditis lasts for only a few weeks. Often, women don't even realize what's wrong with them, because the symptoms are mild and usually associated with the natural fatigue that accompanies taking care of a newborn.

These conditions clear up by themselves. Short-lived Hashimoto's thyroiditis is usually more common than silent thyroiditis after delivery, and, in more severe cases, thyroid hormone is administered temporarily to alleviate the hypothyroid symptoms. Women who experience this sudden thyroid flare-up tend to re-experience it with each pregnancy, however. Obviously, women who do experience postpartum thyroiditis are predisposed to thyroid disorders and seem to be vulnerable in that particular area. Since it's not feasible to screen for this condition in advance, there's really no way to prevent it.

Diagnosing postpartum thyroiditis Today, it should be standard practice for all pregnant women in North America to have their thyroid glands tested after delivery. Regardless of how you feel, request that your doctor perform a thyroid function test within a few days. This is a simple, easy-as-pie blood test. End of story. This test will determine whether you're either over- or underproducing thyroid hormone. If your thyroid test is normal yet you still have symptoms of PPD or maternal blues, then you can rule out a physical cause for your symptoms.

Treating postpartum thyroiditis Most women will experience hypothyroid symptoms (see chapter 2). In this case, you may be monitored and given no medication unless the symptoms are severe enough to warrant it. Medication is one tiny pill that is thyroid replacement hormone: it simply replaces or supplements (determined by your dosage) the thyroid hormone your body makes naturally. Often postpartum thyroiditis resolves on its own.

If you're hyperthyroid symptoms are severe, you may be placed on the antithyroid drug known as propylthiouracil (PTU)—medication that quiets down your thyroid until it corrects itself. Regardless of whether you are given thyroid hormone or PTU, you can still breast-feed safely.

Postpartum Thyroiditis, Blues, or Postpartum Depression?

If you look at the symptoms of hypothyroidism in chapter 2, it's easy to see how they can be confused with symptoms of postpartum depression—especially since fatigue and depression are symptoms of hypothyroidism! That said, it's important not to confuse postpartum depression with maternal blues. Here's an overview:

Your life changes when you have a baby, which often leads to dramatic mood changes: "postpartum blues," which is sometimes confused with postpartum depression. The phrase *postpartum depression,* however, has been used incorrectly by the media, confusing three *separate* psychiatric conditions that occur in the postpartum phase.

Documented mental disturbances following pregnancy have a long history. A connection between depression and pregnancy was recognized as early as 1840. First, normal fatigue and feelings of "letdown," in that you've been excited and preparing for the birth, are common and normal. True postpartum psychological and emotional disturbances range from what's known as "maternal blues" to true *postpartum depression,* where one experiences symptoms ranging from major depression (see chapter 3) to something known as *postpartum psychosis,* the kind of diagnosis made in a situation where a woman loses touch with reality and becomes psychotic, believing, for example, that her newborn is evil or abnormal in some way. Postpartum psychosis occurs in 2 of every 1,000 deliveries, not as uncommon as one is led to believe.

Maternal blues As many as 70 percent of all women will suffer from *maternal blues* after delivery. The maternal blues are common, nothing to worry about, mild and transitory, meaning short-term. This condition usually occurs within the first ten days (averaging three or four days) after delivery.

Symptoms of maternal blues are frequent crying episodes, mood swings, feelings of sadness, low energy, anxiety, insomnia, restlessness, and irritability. Women who experience these feelings should feel comforted that these feelings are normal and will pass. It will last for a couple of weeks.

Maternal blues are most likely caused by enormous hormonal shifts in your body. There is not any real documented proof that what you're feeling is hormonal, however. Since we do know that hormonal shifts definitely cause premenstrual mood swings as well as menopausal mood swings, and we do know that estrogen levels are depleted after childbirth, it's likely that hormones are the culprit.

Nevertheless, there are other causes that have to do with an enormous lifestyle shift. This includes an increase in stress and responsibility, worry about your newborn, physical discomfort associated with your postpartum "physique," and possible exhaustion following labor and delivery.

There is also a kind of "letdown" feeling that some women experience. During pregnancy, there is excitement and anticipation about the big day. Then, the "big day" arrives, you experience an enormous physical strain, and all of the energy and excitement you have invested in the experience needs an emotional outlet. So you cry. Similar feelings tend to follow weddings and big trips. In this case, though, while one kind of adventure is over, another adventure is beginning.

New family conflicts often surface after delivery, too. If this is a first grandchild, the emotional tug-of-war between the two (or more) sets of grandparents may contribute to your stress. And don't forget—baby-naming, baby-naming ceremonies, christenings, baptisms, choosing godparents, circumcision decisions, and "bris" planning all take their toll on your level of stress and can create dismal conflicts that are never settled. This one's hurt; that one's offended; he disapproves; she can't believe you did this or that. You get the idea. Often these family wars interfere with you and your partner's relationship and enjoyment of the newborn.

If you're on maternity leave, your sudden change in daily activities may be a shock to your system, and you may have difficulty adjusting to your new schedule.

And, too often, babies are planned as a way to patch up relationship problems between partners. This can prove to be a mistake.

Unless you're feeling so bad you cannot function at all, give it a couple of weeks and see if you feel any better. If these feelings persist, you should seek out counseling and explore whether your feelings are truly related to your postpartum condition or are perhaps related to other problems that are only now surfacing. Pregnancy can mask relationship problems (that you may not have been aware of) or expose relationship problems. The pregnancy also masks lifestyle ruts that will eventually resurface after delivery. In other words, don't expect old problems to disappear just because you've had a baby.

Postpartum depression (PPD) Postpartum depression is more serious and persistent, and affects 10 to 15 percent of the postpartum population. Depression can begin at any time after delivery—from the first few hours afterward to a few weeks after. These symptoms include sadness, mood changes, lack of energy, loss of interest, change in appetite, fatigue, guilt, self-loathing, suicidal thoughts, and poor concentration and memory. When these feelings last for more than a couple of weeks, the consequences can be truly negative, leading to problems with bonding and relationship trouble. However, women don't go from the "maternal blues" to depression. In fact, you can feel well after delivery and then *suddenly* develop postpartum depression.

The causes of postpartum depression are possibly similar to those cited as causes for the milder maternal blues. But women at risk for this more serious depression are those with a family history of depression and women who have a poor support system at home (spouseless, bad relationship with partner, teenage mothers, and so on).

Interestingly, in some studies, a significant portion of new fathers suffer from an "adjustment disorder" after the arrival of the newborn, sometimes called the "paternal blues." This definitely suggests that the causes are not rooted in hormonal changes but rather lifestyle changes.

Many studies have looked into psychosocial issues revolving around PPD. In one study looking at educated, white, middle-class, married women in their early thirties who returned to work within the first year after delivery, marital adjustment and child-care stress significantly influenced the severity of their PPD symptoms. Those with lower self-esteem and more stress reported more severe PPD symptoms. In fact, mothers with low self-esteem were thirty-nine times more likely to suffer from PPD than those with high self-esteem. Studies on teenage mothers confirm these figures, too. Teen-age mothers typically have more frequent bouts with PPD than adult mothers as a direct result of poor social support systems and lower self-esteem. Inner-city, low-income women developed PPD at double the rate of middle-class women. Not surprisingly, single mothers with no partners were at particular risk for postpartum depression.

Unfortunately, PPD can also affect a baby's temperament during its first year as the baby intuitively responds to the mother's "vibes." The reverse is true, of course, when women are coping with a colicky or difficult baby. Women with PPD who are caring for older children as well as the new baby report feelings of being overwhelmed by their child-care duties. They also report feelings of guilt, loss, and anger as a result. Irrational thinking and robot-like, "going-through-the-motions" actions were common experiences cited in one study.

Treating PPD If you do begin to notice these feelings, treatment is available with a qualified mental health practitioner. You may just need some counseling or to be put on antidepressant medication. Counseling can vary from short-term "sorting out your life" chats (interpersonal therapy) to cognitive behavioral therapy. It really varies depending on the severity of your symptoms. In addition, there are now a number of postpartum support groups where you can talk to other women in the same boat. This is really helpful and may help you to put all of your feelings into a healthier perspective. If you are taking medications for your condition, you should check as to whether or not they are compatible with breast-feeding. (Most anti-depressants prescribed today are just fine, but it's wise to double-check.)

Research shows that women who have experienced postpartum depression at least once have a 30 to 60 percent chance of reexperiencing it with a subsequent pregnancy. As a result, some hospitals are offering antidepressant therapy to women with a history of PPD, utilizing drugs such as nortriptyline. These antidepressants are administered twenty-four hours after delivery for a period of roughly twenty weeks.

When postpartum depression goes untreated, it can have consequences for the baby. Some psychiatrists report that it can interfere with bonding, cognitive, and behavioral development. In some instances, a therapist may suggest that you have some extra help at home until you are "on your feet" again.

Unfortunately, many women who have postpartum thyroiditis are misdiagnosed as having postpartum depression. For these women, a diagnosis of postpartum depression can be enough to ... drive them crazy!

Postpartum psychosis Postpartum psychosis is very serious and requires hospitalization. This affects a very small portion of women and usually begins in the first month after delivery. Basically, this is when you're usually totally out of touch with the world around you. *(Hint: If you're able to read this book, you probably don't have postpartum psychosis.)*

This condition usually indicates other psychiatric disorders, but women can suddenly develop the following psychotic symptoms: delusions that the child is dead or defective, denial that the birth ever took place, or hearing voices (inside their head) that tell them to harm the infant. Accompanying symptoms include sleep disorders, intense confusion, loss of energy, and, hence, difficulty caring for the child. Women at risk for this are those with:

- a past history of a psychotic episode or a past diagnosis of postpartum psychosis
- women who have manic-depressive illness (bipolar disorder)
- women with a family history of bipolar affective psychosis

This is a serious psychiatric illness that needs to be treated with medications and therapies. In some cases, the infant may need to be cared for temporarily by another family member.

Your Baby's Thyroid

The baby's thyroid begins to function somewhere between the tenth and twelfth week of pregnancy. Thyroid hormones are important for the development of the fetal nervous system. The hormones at this stage come primarily from the baby's thyroid gland secretions; only very small amounts of the mother's thyroid hormone cross the placenta.

Iodine in the mother's diet will also cross the placenta and is used by the fetal thyroid gland to make thyroid hormone. Iodine deficiency, on the other hand, can cause newborn hypothyroidism or mental retardation and is a major health problem in underdeveloped countries. But since there is an overabundance of iodine in the North American diet, disorders caused by a lack of dietary iodine don't happen here. (See Table 4.2 for what can cause thyroid disease in your baby.)

Fetal Hypothyroidism

Antithyroid medications, ordinary or nonradioactive iodine, and sometimes maternal thyroid antibodies can cross the placenta and cause hypothyroidism in the baby.

Plain iodine, which is present in medications like some cough syrups, for example, can cause a goiter in the fetus making delivery difficult or causing respiratory obstruction. For this reason, iodine-containing drugs should never be used in pregnancy except in the case of extreme hyperthyroidism—sometimes called "thyroid storm."

Unfortunately, there is no simple blood test to assess the baby's thyroid function in the womb, although measurements of thyroid hormone or TSH levels in the amniotic fluid sac have been used in research studies. Plain X-ray will sometimes show delayed bone development in fetal hypothyroidism, but this test is usually not recommended because the X-ray itself can cause more damage to the fetus than the underlying condition. Screening for hypothyroidism at

TABLE 4.2 Mother and Child and Thyroid Disease

When baby has ...	You may have ...
Fetal hyperthyroidism	Graves' disease (your antibodies crossed the placenta)
Fetal hypothyroidism	Hashimoto's disease (your antibodies crossed the placenta)
	Taken too high a dosage of antithyroid pills
	Taken drugs containing too much iodine
Fetal goiter	A goiter
	Hashimoto's disease
	Taken drugs containing too much iodine
	Taken too high a dosage of antithyroid pills
Neonatal hyperthyroidism	Graves' disease or Hashimoto's disease (your antibodies crossed the placenta)
Neonatal hypothyroidism	A goiter caused by a shortage in iodine
	Hashimoto's disease

Source: Adapted from Patty Westcott, Thyroid Problems: A Practical Guide to Symptoms and Treatment (London: Thorsons/HarperCollins, 1995), 91.

birth—now done routinely in North America on all newborns—is still the best method for determining whether your baby is hypothyroid and whether the infant needs short-term or long-term treatment in the form of thyroid replacement hormone. This is discussed in the next section.

Fetal Hyperthyroidism

When the fetus is hyperthyroid the condition is known as fetal thyrotoxicosis. This happens when maternal thyroid-stimulating antibodies cross the placenta, as in the case of Graves' disease. Fetal hyperthyroidism is unusual, though. In most cases when the mother herself is hyperthyroid and is being treated with antithyroid drugs, the drugs wind up treating the baby as well by crossing the placenta.

However, if the mother's hyperthyroidism occurred in the past and was already treated via radioactive iodine or surgery, she can still have thyroid-stimulating antibodies in her blood even though she's no longer hyperthyroid. Since the mother is well and isn't exhibiting any hyperthyroid symptoms, fetal hyperthyroidism is simply not suspected. When the fetus is hyperthyroid, the fetal heart rate is consistently above the normal limit of 160 beats per minute, and high levels of thyroid-stimulating antibodies will be present in the mother's blood.

All women with Graves' disease or a history of Graves' disease should be tested for thyroid-stimulating antibodies late in pregnancy. The consequences of untreated fetal hyperthyroidism can lead to low birth weight and small head size, fetal distress in labor, neonatal heart failure, and respiratory distress. Putting the mother on antithyroid drugs during pregnancy will treat the baby in this situation, but after delivery it will be necessary to continue treatment for the baby as well as perform follow-up tests. See the section below for more details.

Neonatal or Congenital Hypothyroidism
Roughly 1 in 4,000 babies is born with either neonatal or congenital hypothyroidism. Neonatal hypothyroidism is different from congenital hypothyroidism. In the first case, the baby is born without a thyroid gland. In the second case, the baby is born with what appears to be a normal thyroid gland but then develops symptoms of hypothyroidism after its first twenty-eight days of life; this is known as congenital hypothyroidism which is treated no differently than neonatal hypothyroidism. In this case, while the condition was present at birth, the symptoms didn't manifest until later. Congenital hypothyroidism is just as serious as neonatal hypothyroidism symptoms, and may not be obvious until brain damage has already set in.

Neonatal hypothyroidism or congenital hypothyroidism are very serious conditions that can lead to severe brain damage and developmental impairment. They can occur from an iodine deficiency in the mother's diet. This is common in more remote or mountainous areas of the world where iodine is not readily available. In fact, iodine deficiency is the most common cause of mental retardation in underdeveloped countries. Fortunately, this is not a problem in North

America because most of our salt is iodized. (And low-salt diets still contain enough iodine for our needs.)

Neonatal screening for hypothyroidism The wonderful news is that neonatal screening for hypothyroidism in newborns was introduced in the mid-1970s, and usually catches neonatal hypothyroidism while preventing congenital hypothyroidism from developing. In North America, all babies are given a "heelpad" test approximately two days after birth to check for hypothyroidism.

The heelpad test involves a blood sample taken via a small heel prick and sent to a laboratory for analysis. Usually the test confirms that your baby's thyroid gland is functioning normally. In rare instances, the initial tests may be unclear or "inconclusive." If this happens, the laboratory usually notifies the hospital where your child was born, as well your family physician. Then, someone contacts you to request another blood sample from your baby. If your child is in fact hypothyroid at birth, an endocrinologist and pediatrician will be consulted, and your baby will be given thyroid replacement hormone daily.

As a precaution, before you leave the hospital with your newborn, ask your doctor whether the heelpad test or thyroid test was administered. If for some reason the test was not done, request it, and make certain that you find out the results of the test. If hypothyroidism is diagnosed at birth, any serious consequences are preventable by administering thyroid replacement hormone to the baby. In this case, intellectual and physical growth will be normal.

A Word About Down's Syndrome

At one time, it was believed that fetal or neonatal hypothyroidism caused Down's syndrome. In the nineteenth century, animal thyroid hormone was administered to children with Down's syndrome in the belief that it would normalize their development. We now know that hypothyroidism has absolutely nothing to do with Down's syndrome. Down's syndrome is caused by a chromosomal abnormality in which there is an extra chromosome. For more information, consult my book, *The Pregnancy Sourcebook*.

Neonatal Hyperthyroidism

Hyperthyroidism only occurs in infants born to mothers who are hyperthyroid. Most cases are not reported, and it occurs in 1 of 70 babies born to hyperthyroid mothers. As discussed above, neonatal hyperthyroidism occurs when fetal hyperthyroidism is not caught. Fortunately, this type of hyperthyroidism in a newborn lasts only as long as the mother's antibodies remain in the baby's bloodstream—usually from three to twelve weeks. As well, this condition is usually mild, since most women who are hyperthyroid produce only low levels of thyroid-stimulating antibodies.

Occasionally, if the hyperthyroidism is severe at birth, babies can be born with prominent eyes, irritability (they cry a lot), flushed skin, and a fast pulse—all classic hyperthyroid symptoms. These babies tend to be long and scrawny and, although they have large appetites, may not gain any weight. The cranial bones may also be malformed. Some fetuses die before birth because of this illness, though. Infants who are hyperthyroid are always treated with antithyroid medication; radioactive iodine is never given to infants, and performing a thyroidectomy on an infant is unnecessary since the disease runs its course in eight to twelve weeks. Sometimes plain iodine is used, too.

❧

This chapter is limited to thyroid-related issues involving fertility and pregnancy. It does not cover the myriad issues involving infertility, pregnancy health and nutrition, or breast-feeding issues. For more information, please consult my reproductive health "trilogy": *The Fertility Sourcebook, The Pregnancy Sourcebook,* and *The Breastfeeding Sourcebook.* Thyroid problems continue to interfere with the natural stages of our reproductive cycles. The next chapter discusses how symptoms of menopause can mask a thyroid problem and vice versa.

CHAPTER 5

Thyroid Disease and Menopause

Menopause is a recent phenomenon in our society. Anywhere from sixty to a hundred years ago, women simply died prior to menopause. Only in this century have women ever outlived their ovaries.

Menopause is a Greek term taken from the words *menos,* which means "month," and *pause,* which means "arrest"—the arrest of the menstrual cycle. It is a time in every woman's life when her ovaries are slowing down, running out of eggs, and getting ready to retire. The process involves a complex shutting down of hormones that have nourished the menstrual cycle until this point. As a result, the normal hormonal fluctuations women are used to throughout their menstrual cycles become far more erratic. They are responsible for the infamous "menopausal mood swings" that have created much of the negative mythology surrounding menopause in our culture.

Nevertheless, natural menopause and *menarche* (the first menstrual period) have a lot in common: they are both gradual processes that women ease into. A woman does not suddenly wake up and find herself in menopause any more than a young girl wakes up and finds herself in puberty. However, when menopause occurs surgically—the by-product of an oopherectomy, ovarian failure following a hysterectomy or certain cancer therapies—it can prove an extremely jarring process. *One out of every three women in North America will not make it to the age of sixty with her uterus intact.* These women may indeed wake up one morning to find themselves in menopause and, as a result, will suffer far more noticeable and severe menopausal symptoms than their natural menopause counterparts. It is because of *surgical*

99

menopause that hormonal replacement therapy (HRT) and estrogen replacement therapy (ERT or "unopposed estrogen") have become such hotly debated issues in women's health. The loss of estrogen, in particular, leads to drastic changes in the body's chemistry that trigger a more aggressive aging process (discussed further below).

Women with thyroid disease have a little more to be concerned about than women without thyroid disease. First, estrogen loss increases *all* women's risk of heart disease, which is the major cause of death for postmenopausal women. But in postmenopausal women with thyroid disease, the risk of heart disease may increase as a result of cardiovascular changes due to hyper- or hypothyroidism (see chapter 2). Second, hyperthyroidism can speed the process of osteoporosis, also a risk for women after menopause.

The purpose of this chapter is to discuss both the natural and surgical menopausal facts of life for women with thyroid disease, which include the myths of menopause, the symptoms of menopause, the osteoporosis issue, and the variety of health concerns that women with thyroid disease face as they age. The benefits and risks of HRT (hormone replacement therapy with estrogen and progesterone) and ERT (estrogen replacement therapy given to women who have had hysterectomies) are also discussed. Remember that your age, medical history, and menopausal symptoms all need to be factored into the HRT or ERT decision and weighed against the health risks your thyroid condition poses.

Natural Menopause

When menopause occurs naturally, it tends to take place anywhere between the ages of forty-eight and fifty-two, but it can occur as early as your late thirties, or as late as your mid-fifties. When menopause occurs *before* age forty-five, it is technically considered "early menopause," but, just as menarche is genetically predetermined, so is menopause. For an average woman with an unremarkable medical history, what she eats or does in terms of daily activity will *not* influence the timing of her menopause. Women who have had chemotherapy or been exposed to high levels of radiation (such as radiation therapy in their

Menopause or Thyroid?

The following menopausal symptoms can also be confused with symptoms of hypo- or hyperthyroidism:

- erratic periods
- hot flashes (women who are hyperthyroid will feel "hot" all the time)
- vaginal dryness and/or changes in libido
- muscle aches and pains (could be signs of bone loss)
- skin changes
- irritability
- mood swings

pelvic area for cancer treatment), however, may go into menopause earlier. In any event, the average age of menopause is fifty to fifty-one.

Other causes that have been cited as triggers of early menopause include mumps (in small groups of women, the infection causing the mumps has been known to spread to the ovaries, thus shutting them down prematurely) and women with specific autoimmune diseases such as lupus or rheumatoid arthritis (in some of these women, their bodies develop antibodies to their own ovaries and attack the ovaries).

The Stages of Natural Menopause

Socially, the word *menopause* refers to a process, not a precise moment in the life of your menstrual cycle. But medically, the word *menopause* does indeed refer to one precise moment: the date of your last period. However, the events preceding and following menopause amount to a huge change for women both physically and socially. *Physically,* this process is divided into four stages:

1. *Premenopause:* Although some doctors may refer to a thirty-year-old woman in her childbearing years as "premenopausal," this is not really an appropriate label. The term *premenopause* ideally refers to women on the "cusp" of menopause. Their periods have just *started* to get

irregular, but they do not yet experience any classic menopausal symptoms such as hot flashes or vaginal dryness. A woman in premenopause is usually in her mid-to-late forties. If your doctor says you are premenopausal, you might want to ask how that term is defined.

2. *Perimenopause:* This term refers to women who are in the thick of menopause—their cycles are wildly erratic, and they are experiencing hot flashes and vaginal dryness. This label is applicable for about four years, covering the first two years prior to the official "last" period to the next two years following the last menstrual period. Women who are perimenopausal will be in the age groups discussed above, averaging to about age fifty-one.

3. *Menopause:* This refers to your final menstrual period. You will not be able to pinpoint your final period until you've been completely free from periods for one year. Then, you should count back to the last period you charted, and that date is the date of your menopause. *Important: After more than one year of no menstrual periods, any vaginal bleeding is now considered to be abnormal.*

4. *Postmenopause:* This term refers to the last third of most women's lives: ranging from women who have been free of menstrual periods for at least four years to women celebrating their 100th birthday. In other words, once you're past menopause, you'll be referred to as postmenopausal for the rest of your life. Sometimes, the terms *postmenopausal* and *perimenopausal* are used interchangeably. This is technically inaccurate.

Used in a *social* context, however, nobody really bothers to break down menopause with precision. When you read the phrase *menopausal* in a magazine article, you are reading acceptable medical slang, referring to women who are premenopausal and perimenopausal—a time frame that *includes* the actual menopause. When you read the word *postmenopausal* in a magazine article, you are reading more accepted medical slang, which includes women who are in perimenopause and "official" postmenopause.

"Diagnosing" premenopause or perimenopause When you begin to notice the signs of menopause, discussed next, you will either suspect the approach of menopause on your own or your doctor will put two and two together when you report your "bizarre" symptoms. There are two very simple tests that will accurately determine what's going on and what stage of menopause you're in. Your FSH levels will rise dramatically as your ovaries begin to shut down; these levels are easily checked after one blood test. In addition, your vaginal walls will thin, and the cells lining the vagina will not contain as much estrogen. Your doctor will simply do a Pap-like smear on your vaginal walls—simple and painless—and then analyze the smear to check for vaginal "atrophy"—the thinning and drying out of your vagina. In addition, as I'll discuss below, you need to keep track of your periods and chart them as they become irregular. Your menstrual pattern will be an additional clue to your doctor about whether you are pre- or perimenopausal.

Signs of Natural Menopause

In the past, a long list of hysterical symptoms have been attributed to the "change of life," but medically, there are really just three classic *short-term* symptoms of menopause: erratic periods, hot flashes, and vaginal dryness. All three are caused by a decrease in estrogen. As for the emotional symptoms of menopause, such as irritability, mood swings, melancholy, and so on, they are actually caused by a *rise* in FSH. As the cycle changes and the ovaries' egg supply dwindles, FSH is secreted in very high amounts and reaches a lifetime peak—as much as fifteen times higher; it's the body's way of trying to "jump-start" the ovarian engine. This is why the urine of menopausal women is used to produce human menopausal gonadotropin (HMG), the potent fertility drug that consists of pure FSH.

Every woman entering menopause will experience a change in her menstrual cycle, discussed on page 104. Not all women will experience hot flashes or even notice vaginal changes, however. This is particularly true if a woman is overweight. Estrogen is stored in fat cells, which is why overweight women also tend to be at increased risk for estrogen-dependent cancers. What happens is that the fat cells convert fat into estrogen, creating a type of estrogen reserve that the body will use during menopause, which can reduce the severity of estrogen-loss symptoms.

Erratic periods Every woman will begin to experience an irregular cycle before her last period. Cycles may become longer or shorter with long bouts of amenorrhea. There will also be flow changes, where periods may suddenly become light and scanty, or very heavy and crampy. If you're not entering menopause, you'll need to isolate the cause of your cycle changes, which may indeed indicate a thyroid problem (see chapter 2). But just because you're entering menopause doesn't mean you can't develop a thyroid problem as well.

Hot flashes Roughly 85 percent of all pre- and perimenopausal women experience what is known as "hot flashes." Women suffering from heat intolerance and who feel hot all the time as a result of hyperthyroidism (see chapter 2) may be told that they are having hot flashes when, in fact, they are not. So here's what you need to know about hot flashes.

They can begin when periods are either still regular or have just started to become irregular. The hot flashes usually stop from one to two years after your final menstrual period. A hot flash can feel different for each woman. Some women experience a feeling of warmth in their face and upper body; some women experience hot flashes as simultaneous sweating with chills. Some women feel anxious, tense, dizzy, or nauseous just before the hot flash; some feel tingling in their fingers or heart palpitations. Some women will experience hot flashes during the day. Others will experience them at night and may wake up so wet from perspiration that they need to change their bedsheets and/or night clothes.

Nobody really understands what causes a hot flash, but researchers believe that it has to do with mixed signals from the hypothalamus, which controls both body temperature and sex hormones. Normally, when the body is too warm, the hypothalamus sends a chemical message to the heart to cool off the body by pumping more blood, causing the blood vessels under the skin to dilate, which makes you perspire. During menopause, however, it's believed that the hypothalamus gets confused and sends this "cooling off" signal at the wrong times. A hot flash is not the same as being overheated. Although the skin temparature often rises between 4 to 8 degrees Fahrenheit, the body's internal temperature drops, thus creating this odd sensation. Why does the hypothalamus get so confused? Decreasing levels of estrogen. We know this because when synthetic estrogen is given to replace natural estrogen in the body, hot flashes disappear. Some researchers believe that a decrease in LH is also a key factor, and a variety of other hormones that influence body temperature are being looked at as well. Although hot flashes are harmless in terms of health risks, they are disquieting and stressful symptoms. Certain groups of women will experience more severe hot flashes than others:

- Women who are in surgical menopause (discussed below).
- Women who are thin. When there is less fat on the body to store estrogen reserves, estrogen-loss symptoms are more severe.
- Women who do not sweat easily. An ability to sweat makes extreme temperatures easier to tolerate. Women who have trouble sweating may experience more severe flashes.

Just as you must chart your periods when your cycles become irregular, it's also important to chart your hot flashes. Keep track of when the flashes occur, how long they last, and number their intensity from 1 to 10. This will help you determine a pattern for the flashes and allow you to prepare for them in advance—which will reduce your stress when the flashes begin. It's also crucial to report your hot flashes to your doctor—just as you would any changes in your cycle. Symptoms of hot flashes can also indicate other health problems such as circulatory problems.

What can I do about my hot flashes? Short of taking ERT or HRT, the only thing you can do about your hot flashes is to lessen your discomfort by adjusting your lifestyle to cope with them. The more comfortable you are, the less intense your flashes will feel. Once you establish a pattern by charting the flashes, you can do a few things around the time of day your flashes occur. Some suggestions:

- Avoid synthetic clothing such as polyester because it traps perspiration.
- Use only 100 percent cotton bedding if you have night sweats.
- Avoid clothing with high necks and long sleeves.
- Dress in layers.
- Keep cold drinks handy.
- If you smoke, cut down or quit altogether. Smoking constricts blood vessels and can intensify and prolong a flash. It also leads to complications from thyroid eye disease, discussed in chapter 6.
- Avoid "trigger" foods such as caffeine, alcohol, spicy foods, sugars, and large meals. Substitute herbal teas for coffee or regular tea.
- Discuss the benefits of taking vitamin E supplements with your doctor. Evidence suggests that it is essential for proper circulation and the production of sex hormones.
- Exercise to improve your circulation.
- Reduce your exposure to the sun; sunburn will aggravate your hot flashes because burnt skin cannot regulate heat as effectively. (The sun is discussed further below.)

Vaginal changes Estrogen loss will also cause vaginal changes. Since it is the production of estrogen that causes the vagina to continuously stay moist and elastic through its natural secretions, the loss of estrogen will cause the vagina to become drier, thinner, and less elastic. This may also cause the vagina to shrink slightly in terms of width and length. In addition, the reduction in vaginal secretions causes the vagina to be less acidic. This can put you at risk for more vaginal infections. As a result of these vaginal changes, you will notice a change in your sexual activity. Your vagina may take longer to become lubricated, or you may have to depend on lubricants to have intercourse comfortably.

Estrogen loss can affect other parts of your sex life as well. Your sexual libido may actually increase because testosterone levels can rise when estrogen levels drop. (The general rule is that your levels of testosterone will either stay the same or increase.) However, women who *do* experience an increase in sexual desire will also be frustrated that their vaginas are not accommodating their needs. First, there is the lubrication problem: more stimulation is required to lubricate the vagina naturally. Second, a decrease in estrogen means that less blood flows to the vagina and clitoris, which means that orgasm may be more difficult to achieve or may not last as long as it normally has in the past. Other changes involve the breasts. Normally, estrogen causes blood to flow into the breasts during arousal, which makes the nipples more erect, sensitive, and responsive. Estrogen loss causes less blood to flow to the breasts, which makes them less sensitive. And, finally, because the vagina shrinks as estrogen decreases, it does not expand as much during intercourse, which may make intercourse less comfortable, particularly since it is less lubricated.

Surgical Menopause

Surgical menopause is the result of a bilateral oophorectomy—the removal of both ovaries before natural menopause. Surgical menopause can also be the result of ovarian failure following a hysterectomy or cancer therapy, such as chemotherapy or radiation treatments. A bilateral oophorectomy is often done in conjunction with a hysterectomy or sometimes as a single procedure when, for example, ovarian cancer is suspected.

Bilateral Oophorectomy Symptoms

If you've had your ovaries removed after menopause, you won't be in "surgical menopause." You won't feel any hormonal differences in your body, although you may experience some structural problems. If you've had your ovaries removed before you have reached natural menopause, you'll wake up from your surgery in *post-menopause*. Once the ovaries are removed, your body immediately

stops producing estrogen and progesterone. Your FSH will skyrocket
in an attempt to "make contact" with ovaries that no longer exist.
Unlike women who go through menopause naturally, women wake
up after a bilateral oophorectomy in immediate estrogen "withdrawal." It's that sudden: one day you have a normal menstrual cycle;
the next, you have none whatsoever. This can cause you to become
understandably more depressed, but you'll also feel the physical
symptoms of estrogen loss far more intensely than a woman in natural menopause. That means that your vagina will be *extremely* dry,
your hot flashes will feel like sudden violent heat waves that will be
very disturbing to your system, and, of course, your periods will cease
altogether instead of tapering off naturally. The period that you had
prior to your surgery will have been your last, so you won't even experience pre- or perimenopause, just postmenopause. That means
that you'll need to begin estrogen replacement therapy (ERT) immediately following surgery to prevent these sudden symptoms of
menopause. As discussed below, if you no longer have your uterus,
you'll be on estrogen only, or unopposed estrogen. If you still have
your uterus, you will be placed on estrogen and progesterone hormone replacement therapy (HRT), for the reasons explained in the
HRT/ERT section below. Any short-term menopausal symptoms
will be alleviated by HRT/ERT. Prior to going on HRT/ERT, your
doctor will perform a vaginal smear and blood test to detect your
FSH levels, which will indicate how much estrogen you need.
Dosages will vary from woman to woman, so don't compare notes
with your friends and wonder why "she's taking only X amount"
when you're taking Y amount. ERT and HRT are discussed further
on in the chapter.

If you have just had one ovary removed... If the blood supply leading
to your ovary was not damaged during your surgery, then you should
still be able to produce enough estrogen for your body. If you begin
to go into ovarian failure, the symptoms will depend on how fast the
ovary is failing; you may experience symptoms akin to natural
menopause, or you may experience sudden symptoms mirroring the
surgical menopause experience.

Ovarian Failure Resulting from Cancer Therapy

Chemotherapy and radiation treatments that involve the pelvic area may throw your ovaries into menopause. As described above, you may experience a more gradual menopausal process or be over-whelmed by sudden symptoms of menopause. This will depend on what kind of therapy you've received and the speed at which your ovaries are failing. Before you undergo your cancer treatment, discuss how the treatments will affect your ovaries and what menopausal symptoms you can expect.

Long-Term Effects of Estrogen Loss: Postmenopausal Symptoms

The long-term effects of estrogen loss have to do with traditional symptoms of "aging." One of the key reasons why women will choose HRT or ERT is to slow down or even reverse these symp-toms. Yet it's important to keep in mind that the long-term effects of estrogen loss will not immediately set in after menopause. These changes are subtle and happen over several years. Even women who experience severe menopausal symptoms will not wake up to find that they've suddenly aged overnight; these changes occur gradually whether you experience surgical or natural menopause.

Skin Changes

Skin, like the vagina, tends to lose its elasticity as estrogen decreases; it too becomes thinner because it is no longer able to retain as much water. Sweat and oil glands also produce less moisture, which is what causes the skin to gradually dry, wrinkle, and sag. Skin changes as a result of hypo- or hyperthyroidism (see chapter 2) can be aggravated by skin changes occurring after menopause.

Good moisturizers and skin care will certainly help to keep your skin more elastic, but there is one known factor that aggravates and speeds up your skin's natural aging process, damaging the skin even more: the sun. If you reduce your exposure to the sun, you can dramatically reduce visible aging of your skin. Period. The bad news is that much of the sun's damage to our skin is cumulative over many years. In fact, many researchers believe that when it comes to visible signs of aging, *estrogen loss is only a small factor.* For example, it's known that ultraviolet rays break down collagen and elastin fibers in the skin, which cause it to break down and sag. This is also what puts us at risk for skin cancer, the most notorious of which is melanoma, one of the most aggressive and malignant of all cancers.

Other sun-related problems traditionally linked to estrogen loss are what we call "liver spots"—light brown or tan splotches that develop on the face, neck, and hands as we age. First, these spots have *nothing* to do with the liver; they are sun spots and are caused by sun exposure. In fact, they are sometimes the result of HRT, known in this case as *hyperpigmentation.* Sun spots can also be confused with vitiligo—patches of pigmentation loss—which is a sign of hyper- and hypothyroidism.

Currently, dermatologists are recommending sunblocks having a minimum SPF of 15. In fact, sun damage is so widespread in our population today that sunblock has most likely become part of many North American women's daily cosmetic routine; many women put it on as regularly as a daily moisturizer.

Women struggling with a thyroid disorder may find that their skin is drier and more scaly, while vaginal dryness may be more severe. They may also notice that their nails are deteriorating more rapidly.

The Osteoporosis Issue

Osteoporosis literally means "porous bones" and is perhaps the most feared condition in the postmenopausal community. Unfortunately, osteoporosis is not always preventable and is a classic symptom of aging. Normally in the life of a healthy, unremarkable woman, by her late thirties and forties her bones become less dense. By the time she reaches her fifties, she may begin to experience bone loss in her teeth and become more susceptible to wrist fractures. Gradually, the bones in her spine weaken, fracture, and compress, causing upper back curvature and loss of height, known as a "dowager's hump." Osteoporosis is unfortunately more common in women because, when their skeletal growth is completed, they typically have 15 percent lower bone mineral density and 30 percent less bone mass than a man of the same age. Studies also show that women lose more trabecular bone (the inner, spongy part comprising the internal support of the bone) at a higher rate than men.

Women are prone to three types of osteoporosis: postmeno-pausal, senile, and secondary. Postmenopausal osteoporosis usually develops ten to fifteen years after the onset of menopause. In this case, estrogen loss interferes with calcium absorption, and you begin to lose what is known as your trabecular bone three times faster than the normal rate of trabecular bone loss. You will also begin to lose parts of your cortex (the bone's outer shell)—but not as quickly as the trabecular bone.

Senile osteoporosis affects men and women. It causes you to lose cortical and trabecular bone because of a decrease in bone cell activity that results from aging. Hip fractures are seen most often with this kind of osteoporosis. The decrease in bone cell activity affects your capacity to rebuild bone in the first place. It is also aggravated by low calcium intake.

Secondary osteoporosis means that there is an underlying condition that has caused bone loss. These conditions include chronic renal disease, hypogonadism (an overstimulation of the sex glands—gonads), hyperthyroidism (an overactive thyroid gland), some forms of cancer, gastrectomy (removal of parts of the intestine that interfere with calcium absorption), and the use of anticonvulsants.

Right now, one-and-a-half million Canadians are affected by osteoporosis; 1 in 4 are women over age fifty.

Fracture statistics At least thirty million North American women over age forty-five are affected by osteoporosis, while more than 500,000 postmenopausal women in the U.S. each year will suffer an osteoporosis-related fracture. These fractures usually involve the spine, hip, or distal radius. Fractures will lead to death 12 to 20 percent of the time as a result of pneumonia. As the rib cage moves forward toward the pelvis, gastrointestinal and respiratory problems will increase. Meanwhile, at least 23 percent of all fractures lead to permanent disability after one year. Osteoporosis-related fractures of the wrist, usually the result of a fall on the outstretched hand, are painful and can require a cast for four to six weeks.

Women with thyroid disease, who are suffering from tremors, muscle weakness, or vision problems are also more likely to fall and suffer a fracture.

What causes bone loss anyway? Our bones are always regenerating (known as "remodeling"). This process helps to maintain a constant level of calcium in the blood, which is essential for a healthy heart, blood circulation, and blood clotting. About 99 percent of all the body's calcium is in the bones and teeth; when blood calcium drops below a certain level, the body will take calcium from the bones to replenish it. But by the time we reach our late thirties, our bones lose calcium faster than it can be replaced. The pace of bone calcium loss speeds up for "freshly postmenopausal" women, who are three to seven years beyond menopause. The pace then slows once again, but as we age, the body is less able to absorb calcium from food. One of the most influential factors concerning bone loss is estrogen; it slows or even halts the loss of bone mass by improving our absorption of calcium from the intestinal tract, which allows us to maintain a higher level of calcium in our blood. And the higher the calcium levels in the blood, the less chance you have of losing calcium from your bones to replenish your calcium blood levels. In men, testosterone does the same thing for them regarding calcium absorption, but, unlike women, men never reach a particular age when their testes stop producing testosterone. If they did, they would be just as prone to osteoporosis as women.

But estrogen alone cannot prevent osteoporosis. There is a long list of other factors that affect bone loss. One of the most obvious factors is calcium in our diet. Calcium is regularly lost to urine, feces, and dead skin. We need to continuously account for this loss in our diet. In fact, the less calcium we ingest, the more we force our body to take it out of our bones. Exercise also greatly affects bone density; the more we exercise, the stronger our bones become. In fact, the bone mass we have in our late twenties and early thirties will affect our bone mass at menopause.

Finally, there are several physical conditions and external factors that help to weaken our bones, contributing to bone loss later in life. These include:

- *heavy caffeine and alcohol intake*—because they are diuretics they cause you to lose more calcium in your urine
- *smoking*—research shows that smokers tend to go into menopause earlier, while older smokers have 20 to 30 percent less bone mass than nonsmokers
- *women in surgical menopause who are not on ERT*—losing estrogen earlier than you naturally would have increases bone loss
- *antacids with aluminum and corticosteroids*
- *diseases of the small intestine, liver, and pancreas*—prevents the body from absorbing adequate amounts of calcium from the intestine
- *lymphoma, leukemia, and multiple myeloma*
- *chronic diarrhea from ulcerative colitis or Crohn's disease*— causes calcium loss through feces
- *surgical removal of part of the stomach or small intestine*— affects absorption
- *hypercalciuria*—a condition where one loses too much calcium in the urine
- *early menopause (before age forty-five)*—the earlier you stop producing estrogen, the more likely you are to lose calcium
- *lighter complexions*—women with darker pigments have roughly 10 percent more bone mass than fairer women because they produce more calcitonin, the hormone that strengthens bones
- *low weight*—women with less body fat store less estrogen, which makes the bones less dense to begin with, and more vulnerable to calcium loss
- *women with eating disorders (yo-yo dieting, starvation diets, binge/purge eaters)*—when there is not enough calcium in the bloodstream from our diet, the body will go to the bones to get what it needs. These women also have lower weight
- *a family history of osteoporosis*—studies show that women

born to mothers with spinal fractures have lower bone
mineral density in the spine, neck, and mid-shaft
- *high-protein diet*—contributes to a loss of calcium in urine
- *women who have never been pregnant*—they have not
  experienced the same bursts of estrogen in their bodies as
  women who have been pregnant
- *antacids with aluminum*—they interfere with calcium
  absorption
- *lactose intolerance*—since so much calcium is in dairy foods,
  this allergy is a significant risk factor
- *teenage pregnancy*—when a woman is pregnant in her teens,
  her bones are not yet fully developed, and she can lose as
  much as 10 percent of her bone mass unless she has an
  adequate calcium intake of roughly 2,000 mg during the
  pregnancy, and 2,200 mg while breast-feeding
- *scoliosis*

Thyroid Disease and Osteoporosis

One of the most common questions that women taking thyroid hormone ask is: What is the link between thyroid disease and osteoporosis? Contrary to what most women think, the link has *nothing* to
do with calcitonin, which the thyroid also produces (discussed in
chapter 1). So ladies, here's the real story to set the record straight.

Again, thyroid hormone is something our body uses literally from
head to toe. In general, anyone with too much thyroid hormone
in their system is vulnerable to bone loss. That is because thyroid
hormone will "speed up" or "slow down" bone cells just as it will
speed or slow other processes in our bodies, such as our metabolism.
Osteoblasts are the cells responsible for building bone, while osteoclasts are cells that remove old bone so that the new bone can be replaced. When you are hyperthyroid, osteoclasts get overstimulated; in
short, they go nuts. They begin to remove bone faster than it can be
replaced by the osteoblasts, which are not affected by hyperthyroidism. The result? You wind up with too much bone removed and
subsequent bone loss.

Once your hyperthyroidism is treated, however, and your thyroid hormone replacement medication is balanced, the risk is gone. But, as we all know, finding the right dosage can be tricky, especially since our thyroid hormone dosage requirements change as we age, as we gain or lose weight, and so on. What experts recommend is to make sure you have your thyroid hormone levels checked every year so that you can adjust your dosage accordingly. Women who have had a thyroidectomy to treat thyroid cancer need to be on a slightly higher dosage of thyroid hormone to suppress all thyroid stimulating hormone (TSH) activity. This means that dosage balancing can be especially challenging. What I recommend in all cases—particularly in this one—is to *insist* that your doctor prescribe a thyroid hormone tablet with *precise dosing*—as most of the brand-name tablets offer such as Synthroid®, Levoxyl®, Levothroid®, or Eltroxin® (in Canada only). Some women may do better on 137 mcg instead of 125 or 150 mcg , for example.

To prevent osteoporosis, get your thyroid problem or thyroid dosage under control as quickly as possible. Second, if you have no history of breast cancer, consider going on hormone replacement therapy (HRT). HRT not only halts bone loss but also protects you from heart disease—which claims more women's lives than any other illness. Third, eat well and exercise. Calcium *can* be eaten; exercise *will* build bone mass. See chapter 7 for details on nutrition; it includes the appropriate amount of calcium for women at all stages of their lives.

What If I Cannot Be on HRT?

There are now a host of osteoporosis drugs designed to prevent bone loss. One of them, Evista®, developed by Eli Lilly, seems to have the added benefit of reducing the risk of invasive breast cancer in postmenopausal women.

That said, diet and exercise can really work wonders. It's not enough to just take calcium supplements or eat high-calcium foods; you need to cut down on foods that have diuretic qualities to them: caffeine and alcohol. How much is "enough" calcium? According to the National Institutes of Health Consensus Panel on Osteoporosis, premenopausal women require roughly 1,000 mg of calcium per day; for perimenopausal or postmenopausal women already on HRT or

ERT 1,000 mg; and for peri- and postmenopausal women not taking estrogen, roughly 1,500 mg per day. For women who have already been diagnosed with osteoporosis, the panel recommends 2,500 mg of calcium a day. Foods that are rich in calcium include all dairy products (an 8-oz. glass of milk contains 300 mg calcium), fish, shellfish, oysters, shrimp, sardines, salmon, soybeans, tofu, broccoli, and dark green vegetables (except spinach, which contains oxalic acid, preventing calcium absorption). It's crucial to determine how much calcium you are getting in your diet *before* you start taking any calcium supplements; too much calcium can cause kidney stones in people who are at risk for them. In addition, not all supplements have been tested for absorbency. It's crucial to remember that a calcium supplement is, in fact, a supplement, and should not replace a high-calcium diet. Thus, the dosage of your supplement would only need to be roughly 400 to 600 mg per day, while your diet should account for the remainder of your 1,000 to 1,500 mg daily intake of calcium. Calcium is discussed more thoroughly in chapter 7.

As for exercise, the best kind of activities are walking, running, biking, aerobic dance, or cross-country skiing. These are considered good ways to put more stress on the bones, thus increasing their mass. Carrying weights is also a good way to increase bone mass.

The most accurate way to measure your risk of osteoporosis is by undergoing bone densitometry (or "DEXA"), which measures bone mass and provides you with a "fracture risk estimate." This test involves low-dose X-ray and takes about thirty minutes. For more information about osteoporosis, see the resource list at the back of this book.

Hormone Replacement Therapy and Thyroid Disease

The average North American woman will live until age seventy-eight, meaning that she will live one-third of her life after menopause. Since women are more prone to heart disease as a result of estrogen loss after menopause, and thyroid disease can dramatically affect the heart (see chapter 2), discuss with your doctor whether hormone replacement therapy is an option for you after menopause. The risk of os-teoporosis also increases if you have suffered hyperthyroidism, which means that, for you, HRT may have even greater benefit. Right now, the Women's Health Initiative (WHI) is studying 25,000 post-menopausal women, many of whom may be affected by thyroid dis-ease as well. The results of this study (expected by 2003) are expected to present concrete facts regarding the perceived benefits of HRT on postmenopausal women experiencing a myriad of other health problems.

Many women, of course, will also be concerned about their risk of breast cancer. Taking estrogen can stimulate or trigger the growth of an estrogen-dependent breast cancer cell (that is, a breast cancer cell that "feeds," or thrives on, the hormone estrogen). Current stud-ies show that these type of cancers are far more treatable than other kinds of breast cancers, but more women die from heart attacks than breast cancer after menopause. The risk of dying from a heart attack may be increased if you suffered damage to your heart as a result of prolonged and untreated hyper- or hypothyroidism. So the thought of preventing heart disease, as well as fractures from osteoporosis, is considered to be a benefit for postmenopausal women with thyroid disease. Nevertheless, you have some thinking to do if you are con-sidering hormone replacement therapy. Here are the facts you need to make a more informed choice.

What Is HRT?

Hormone replacement therapy (HRT) refers to estrogen *and* pro-gesterone; the progesterone is given after menopause to women who still have their uterus to prevent the lining from overgrowing and becoming cancerous. Estrogen replacement therapy (ERT) refers to estrogen only, which is given after surgical menopause to women who no longer have a uterus. Both HRT and ERT are "prophylactic" therapy and a "cure" for menopausal symptoms. They are designed to replace the estrogen lost after menopause, and hence:

1. Prevent or even reverse the long-term consequences of estrogen loss (osteoporosis, skin changes, vaginal thinning and dryness, and a list of other ailments).

2. Treat the short-term symptoms of menopause such as the hot flashes and vaginal dryness.

Therefore, you have the choice of taking HRT or ERT as either a short-term or long-term therapy. There are also some risks involved with HRT and ERT that you will need to weigh against the benefits, however.

The Benefits

What exactly is estrogen responsible for in our bodies? In addition to protecting our bones and maintaining our reproductive organs, estrogen also helps to maintain appropriate levels of high-density lipoprotein (HDL), which keeps our arteries clear of plaque and prevents them from clogging and causing heart attacks and strokes. By raising HDL, known as the "good cholesterol," the "bad cholesterol," the low-density lipoproteins that cause fatty substances to collect in the arteries (causing arteriosclerosis), drop. Estrogen also helps to protect us from rheumatoid arthritis. It is our ovaries, of course, that make estrogen, but other sources of estrogen come from androstenedione (a hormone) and testosterone, which are converted by our tissues into a form of estrogen called *estrone,* a weaker form of estrogen than the kind our ovaries produce. Obese women have estrogen in greater amounts. Although this may prevent any severe menopausal symptoms, estrone is *not* considered a potent enough form of estrogen to protect against osteoporosis or heart disease.

Thirty years ago, all women, regardless of whether they still had a uterus, were placed on pure estrogen hormone without any progesterone. This is known as "unopposed estrogen therapy" because in a natural cycle the progesterone "opposes" the estrogen and counterbalances high estrogen levels. It prevents you from becoming "estrogen toxic" at far higher dosages than what is given today. This created several problems. First, women experienced side effects similar to the early oral contraceptives: nausea, dizziness, bloating, etc. Second, women who went into menopause naturally tended to develop endometrial hyperplasia (overgrowth of the uterine lining), which often became uterine cancer. Finally, both surgical and natural menopause recipients of this estrogen therapy were considered at higher risk of developing estrogen-dependent cancers, such as breast cancer and ovarian cancer.

Today, all women who have gone through menopause naturally and decide to go on HRT will be given estrogen *and* progesterone. The progesterone, of course, triggers the uterine lining to shed regularly, *which prevents endometrial hyperplasia,* which is what predisposed women on unopposed estrogen (i.e., those with a uterus, taking only estrogen) to develop uterine cancer. Estrogen and progesterone *together* also mirror the normal menstrual cycle and help prevent the side effects normally felt from taking estrogen alone. Estrogen levels are today much lower than they were in the past; current HRT doses are about ten times lower than the average combination oral contraceptive.

If you are in surgical menopause, you will not need any progesterone because you are no longer at risk for endometrial hyperplasia. But because your menopausal symptoms will be more severe, your need for estrogen may be greater. Again, however, since today's estrogen doses are much lower, you will likely not experience any short-term side effects from taking it.

What to expect in the short term Generally, HRT/ERT will begin to relieve your estrogen-loss menopausal symptoms within days of starting the therapy. Your hot flashes will disappear, your vagina will become moist again and will lubricate on its own during sex, and your vagina's acidic environment will be restored, preventing yeast and other vaginal infections from plaguing you. However, if you change your mind and discontinue the therapy, your symptoms will return in a far more severe form.

What to expect in the long term Your HDL levels will be maintained, and you will not experience severe bone loss, which can put you at risk for fractures and breakages. However, research shows that HRT is more effective than ERT in preventing osteoporosis.

As for heart disease, roughly half a million North American women die of heart disease every year. Heart attack statistics are much lower in premenopausal women than in postmenopausal women. In the premenopause age group, men outperform women by a vast degree. However, ten to fifteen years after menopause, women equal men in number of heart attacks. To date, most of the research indicates that estrogen will protect women from heart disease.

But it's also important to review these studies in the proper context. First, the women selected for these studies are generally upper middle-class and educated, two major factors that appear to decrease the risk of heart disease anyway. Second, women who take estrogen are usually healthier and more willing to make other lifestyle changes that will lower their risk—such as maintaining a proper diet or not smoking.

Finally, some animal research revealed that the progesterone added to HRT may have the *opposite* influence on HDL compared to estrogen. What you might want to do if you decide to go on HRT for strictly the heart benefit is to have your cholesterol level checked before you start HRT—as a "baseline," and then get your levels checked after you're on HRT for about three months. If there is no improvement in your cholesterol levels, you may want to review your decision with your doctor.

The heart benefits experienced with estrogen hold true only if the estrogen is taken orally, not in patches or vaginal creams. In order for estrogen to work its magic with HDL, it needs to be metabolized in the liver.

Finally, estrogen will not counteract a poor diet and lifestyle. If you smoke, drink excessively, are under tremendous stress, eat copious amounts of the wrong foods (see chapter 7), or have a family history of heart attack, do not expect estrogen alone to shield you from heart disease.

The Risks

The risk that once was the chief concern regarding estrogen use is uterine cancer. Today, it is no longer a risk! In the past, unopposed estrogen was given both to women who still *had* a uterus and women who did not. Of course, if you do not have a uterus, there is no risk of uterine cancer. But what about women who had one? Well, a funny thing happened: doctors *forgot* about the uterus, ignoring the fact that the female body is very smart. When it detects estrogen in the body, it says: "Oh, look—estrogen again! Better start preparing the endometrium for a baby!" And guess what? There's no progesterone to trigger the lining to begin shedding, and certainly no baby—so the lining just keeps growing until you wind up with endometrial hyperplasia, overgrowth of the uterine lining, and, eventually, uterine cancer. When the uterine cancer rate began to increase among uterus "owners" on unopposed estrogen, the medical community realized its mistake, remembered the uterus and the importance of progesterone, and today *will not administer unopposed estrogen to any woman with a uterus.*

The Forms of HRT and ERT

You can take estrogen in a number of ways. The most common estrogen product uses a synthesis of various estrogens that are derived from the urine of pregnant horses. That way the estrogen will mimic nature more accurately. Estrogen replacement comes in either pills, patches (transdermal), or vaginal creams. Other common, synthetic forms of estrogen include micronized estradiol, ethinyl estradiol, esterified estrogen, and quinestrol.

As short-term therapy, you may only need the vaginal cream to help with vaginal dryness or bladder problems. For long-term therapy, you'll need the pill form if you want to protect yourself from heart disease. Premarin® comes under a variety of brand names, each just as good as the other. Estrogen can also be "worn." In this case, it's placed in a small plastic patch approximately the size of a silver dollar, worn on the abdomen, thighs, or buttocks, and changed twice weekly.

When estrogen is in patch or cream form, it goes directly to the bloodstream—bypassing the liver—and hence does not affect HDL or protect against heart disease. Some women also have an allergic reaction to the skin patch and get a rash. If you're one of them, you should investigate taking estrogen in other forms.

Finally, you can also take estrogen injections. Each shot lasts from three to six weeks, though it is expensive and inconvenient because the dosages are not as flexible.

Women react differently to Premarin or other synthetic forms of estrogen; some do better than others on different chemical recipes. So if you don't do well on Premarin, for example, see if estradiol is better for you, or vice versa. Don't just give up and go off HRT or ERT altogether; explore all the possibilities. Dosages are discussed below.

Progesterone Synthetic progestins (a family of progesterone drugs that include natural progesterone) are norethindrone or norethindrone acetate. Natural progestin is medroxyprogesterone.

Progestins are taken in separate tablets along with estrogen. Together, the estrogen and progestin you take is called HRT. HRT can be administered in two ways: cyclically or continuously. Taking HRT cyclically is very similar to taking an oral contraceptive because the hormones more closely mirror a natural cycle. The first day you start is considered day "1" of your mock "cycle." You take estrogen from day 1 to 25; you then add the progesterone from day 14 to 25. Then you stop all pills and bleed for two or three days—just as you would on a combination OC. This vaginal bleeding is called "withdrawal bleeding," which is lighter and shorter than a normal menstrual period. It lasts only two or three days—just like a period on a combination OC. In fact, if the bleeding is heavy or prolonged for some reason, this is a warning that something is not right, and you should have it checked.

In addition, you may experience "breakthrough bleeding"— spotting during the first three weeks after you begin HRT. This kind of bleeding is, again, similar to what happens on a combination OC. This bleeding usually goes away after a few months, but report it anyway. You may need to switch to a lower dose of estrogen or take a higher dose of your progestin. Once your mini-period of withdrawal bleeding is finished, you simply start the cycle again. Many women cannot tolerate cyclical HRT because they feel as though they should be rid of their periods by now and not have to deal with pads and tampons ever again. However, it is believed that cyclical HRT offers slightly better heart protection.

When HRT is taken continuously, you simply take one estrogen pill and one progestin pill each day. Taken this way, the progesterone counteracts the estrogen; no uterine lining is built up, so there is no withdrawal bleeding that needs to happen.

The appropriate dosages Every woman requires a different dosage of estrogen and progestin. But you will always be placed on the *lowest* possible dosage of either one and may have the dosage increased gradually if necessary. If your estrogen dosage is too high, you'll experience side effects similar to oral contraceptives: headaches, bloating, etc. Before you determine how much estrogen you will need, it is crucial to determine first how much your body is still producing; this really depends on your weight, menopausal symptoms, and a hundred other things.

Common side effects If you are taking *cyclical* progestins with your estrogen because you still have your uterus, bleeding is *not* a side effect! The whole point of adding progestin to your estrogen is to trigger withdrawal bleeding and for your uterine lining to shed routinely. However, if you are taking continuous progestins with your estrogen, bleeding is not normal and should be checked into.

Common side effects of estrogen will include fluid retention because estrogen will decrease the amount of salt and water excreted by the kidneys, which is retained by legs, breasts, and feet, all of which can swell. You may weigh more due to the fluid retention and might also gain weight. Nausea is another common side effect also seen with OCs. This happens during the first two or three months of your therapy and should just disappear on its own. Some women find that taking their dosages at night (for pills) may remedy this. Decreasing the dosage is also an option.

Some other side effects reported include headaches, skin color changes called *melasma* on the face, more cervical mucous secretion, liquid secretion from breasts, change in curvature of the cornea, jaundice, loss of scalp hair, and itchiness. Again, these side effects vary and depend on the brand you are taking, the dosage, your medical history, and so on.

Are You an HRT or ERT Candidate?

Again, HRT or ERT is not for everyone. Some women make better candidates than others. Here is a guide that may help you to make the decision:

- Do you suffer from severe hot flashes that do not respond to natural remedies, outlined above?
- Are your vaginal changes causing painful intercourse, urinary tract infections, or vaginitis that does not respond to natural remedies, such as more stimulation of the clitoris during sex or sexual lubricants?
- Are you in a high-risk category for endometrial cancer? If so, taking progestin to trigger withdrawal bleeding will lower your risk.
- Are you in a high-risk group for heart attacks or strokes? If so, ERT or HRT will lower your risk.
- Are you in a high-risk group for developing osteoporosis? Again, ERT or HRT will lower your risk.

Women who should not be on ERT or HRT

- Women with (a history of) endometrial cancer should not be on unopposed estrogen ERT. Again, if you still have a uterus you will be placed on HRT (estrogen and progesterone), which lowers your cancer risk anyway.
- Women with breast cancer. This is in debate. See page 129.
- Women who have had a stroke. Neither ERT or HRT is recommended.
- Women who have a blood-clotting disorder. Neither ERT or HRT is recommended.
- Women with undiagnosed vaginal bleeding. Neither therapy is recommended.
- Women with liver dysfunction. You can be on the estrogen patch or vaginal cream to relieve your menopausal symptoms, but you should not take any pills orally.

Women who may benefit more from HRT or ERT

Women with thyroid disease are encouraged to discuss whether they are candidates for

HRT, given its protective effects against osteoporosis and heart disease. You may need to think twice if you have the following other conditions, however:

- sickle cell disease
- high blood pressure
- migraines
- uterine fibroids
- a history of benign breast conditions such as cysts or fibroadenomas
- endometriosis
- seizures
- gallbladder disease
- a family history of breast cancer
- a past or current history of smoking

Phytoestrogens: The HRT Alternative

If you are uncomfortable with the idea of taking hormone replacement therapy, you may wish to consider the therapeutic benefits of phytoestrogens, or plant estrogens. Women are treating their symptoms with capsules of powdered herbs such as licorice, burdock, wild yam, motherwort, and dong quai (a.k.a. *Angelica sinensis*).

These herbs contain a multitude of chemicals including estrogenic substances. Although phytoestrogens have been used in Asian cultures for centuries to treat hot flashes, they are just beginning to catch on in the West. The first controlled trial began in 1996 at Columbia-Presbyterian Medical Center in New York.

Many food sources, such as tofu and soy, contain such high concentrations of phytoestrogens that scientists believe they may account for the incredible lack of menopausal symptoms in Japan, which has a soy-heavy diet. Blood levels of phytoestrogens are ten to forty times higher in Japanese women than their Western counterparts, but Japanese women report hot flashes about one-sixth as often as Western women. Even the average vegetarian would not consume nearly as much soy as the average Japanese woman.

Of even more interest, plant hormones not only help to prevent menopausal symptoms but also may protect you from breast cancer;

breast cancer rates are dramatically lower in Japan than in the U.S., but there may be other factors involved, such as childbearing habits and low-fat diets. After menopause, high-fat diets can increase your risk of heart attack and stroke—no matter how much estrogen you take. Meanwhile, bad habits such as coffee, alcohol, and smoking can all increase your risk of osteoporosis. Right now, most doctors will tell you to go ahead and add as much soy as you want to your diet. It may well help; it certainly can't hurt.

What Are the Drawbacks?

Licorice root will increase your blood pressure if you already have hypertension, while wild yam occasionally causes gastrointestinal cramps. Moreover, many people have allergic reactions to a variety of herbs. Finally, because herbal products are not regulated, there is a danger of misuse, overuse, or using poor quality merchandise.

Phytoestrogens can be taken orally or even in cream form, which can be applied to your body parts. Creams are "quasi-natural," however, because the plant hormones they contain are modified in a laboratory. One good question many women are asking is whether phytoestrogens carry the same risks as HRT.

Because plant-based hormones contain chemicals that are similar—but not identical—to your natural estrogen, questions remain about their use.

Other Postmenopausal Concerns

As you age, there are several health problems that might plague you as a result of estrogen loss. But the two primary concerns women need to think about are their risks of heart disease and breast cancer. Following is a brief overview.

Concerns About Heart Disease

Ladies, if you have thyroid disease, you must educate yourselves about the signs and symptoms of heart disease. Again, heart disease kills more postmenopausal women than lung cancer or breast cancer because estrogen loss increases the risk of coronary artery disease. Other risk factors such as smoking, high blood pressure, high cholesterol, obesity, and an inactive lifestyle will further increase your risk. In fact, the Nurses' Health Study, a study involving 120,000 middle-aged women, found that women who were obese had a two- to threefold increase in heart disease, particularly in women with "apple-shaped" figures (meaning abdominal or upper body fat).

Studies indicate that hormone replacement therapy, cholesterol-lowering drugs, and lifestyle changes can significantly reduce the risk of heart disease. Women who are physically active have a 60 to 75 percent lower risk of heart disease than inactive women.

Women and heart disease Heart disease is currently the number-one cause of death in postmenopausal women; more women die of heart disease than lung cancer or breast cancer. Half of all North Americans who die from heart attacks each year are women.

One of the reasons for such high death rates from heart attacks among women is medical ignorance: most studies examining heart disease excluded women (see Introduction), which led to a myth that more men than women die of heart disease. The truth is, more men die of heart attacks before age fifty, while more women die of heart attacks after age fifty as a direct result of estrogen loss. Moreover, women who have had oophorectomies (removal of the ovaries) prior to natural menopause increase their risk of a heart attack by up to *eight times*. Because more women work outside the home than ever before, a number of experts cite stress as a huge contributing factor to increased rates of heart disease in women.

Another problem is that women have different symptoms than men when it comes to heart disease, and so the "typical" warning signs we know about in men—angina, or chest pains—are often never present in women. In fact, chest pains in women are almost never related to heart disease. For women, the symptoms of heart disease, and even an actual heart attack, can be much more vague and seemingly unrelated to heart problems. Signs of heart disease in women include surprising symptoms, some of which may be masked by thyroid problems. A woman experiencing some of these symptoms may be worried she is having a heart attack, when in fact it is purely thyroid related. So, please review the following list carefully.

- Shortness of breath and/or fatigue
- Jaw pain (often masked by arthritis and joint pain)
- Pain in the back of the neck (often masked by arthritis or joint pain)
- Pain down the right or left arm
- Back pain (often masked by arthritis and joint pain)
- Sweating—have your thyroid checked; this is a classic sign of an overactive thyroid gland; also test your blood sugar— you may be low
- Fainting
- Palpitations—again, have your thyroid checked, also a classic symptom of an overactive thyroid
- Bloating (after menopause, would you believe this is a sign of coronary artery blockage?)
- Heartburn, belching, or other gastrointestinal pain (this is often a sign of an actual heart attack in women)
- Chest "heaviness" between the breasts (this is how women experience "chest pain"; some describe it as a "sinking feeling" or burning sensation). Also described as an "aching, throbbing, or squeezing sensation"; "hot poker tab between the chest"; or feeling like your heart jumps into your throat.
- Sudden swings in blood sugar
- Vomiting
- Confusion

Clearly, there are many other causes for the symptoms on this list. But it is important that your doctor includes heart disease as a possible cause, rather than dismissing it because your symptoms are not "male" (which your doctor may refer to as "typical").

Diagnostic tests that can confirm heart disease in women include a physical exam (doctor examining you with a stethoscope); an electrocardiogram; an exercise stress test; an echocardiogram; and a myriad of imaging tests that may use radioactive substances to take pictures of the heart.

If you are diagnosed with heart disease, the "cure" is prevention through diet (see chapter 7), exercise (see page 145), and protection through hormone replacement therapy (see page 116).

Concerns About Breast Cancer

As you probably know, postmenopausal breast cancer is considered to be epidemic among women over fifty. There are many reasons for this, all of which are discussed in my book, *The Breast Sourcebook*. Women at risk for heart disease will probably be told that they should consider hormone replacement therapy to reduce their risk of heart disease, a disease to which they are two to three times more likely to suffer from than the average woman. Therefore, you may be concerned about breast cancer risk and HRT.

It's still not clear whether hormone replacement therapy (HRT) increases your risk of breast cancer, but there's actually more consensus in the medical research community over this issue than many others. That's because the incidence of breast cancer in Western nations rises dramatically anyway after menopause—whether you're on HRT or not. So it's not clear whether HRT really contributes to this increase. The current thinking seems to be that if you're on HRT, there's a slight increased risk of developing breast cancer. But this seems to be because if you do develop it, it's apparently a very treatable type of cancer that's estrogen-receptor positive, meaning that your risk of dying from breast cancer is *decreased*.

If you add up all the data, you may want to rethink HRT if your risk of breast cancer is significant (due to other factors such as family history, for example) or if the risk of breast cancer significantly outweighs your risk of heart disease. For the record, heart disease kills more women than breast cancer, and HRT can definitely lower your cholesterol levels, lower your risk of heart disease, and lower your risk of dying from heart disease. Furthermore, if you are at greater risk for osteoporosis as a result of thyroid disease, HRT stops bone loss. In fact, if begun in the first few years after menopause, HRT will even increase bone mass. Remember: hip and spinal fractures can be very debilitating (often life-threatening) and can truly affect quality of life.

As you can see, many symptoms of estrogen loss can mask, or aggravate, a thyroid problem. Your body's requirements for thyroid hormone also change after menopause. So if you were prescribed thyroid hormone ten years ago, you'll want to revisit your dosage as you approach menopause. Finally, be sure to incorporate some physical activity into your life. Exercise will help reduce your risk of heart disease, breast cancer, and osteoporosis. It will also help you to cope with the symptoms of thyroid disease, such as weight gain, fatigue, and depression. Finally, changes in hormones not only lead to vaginal dryness but also to dry, irritated eyes—a symptom also associated with thyroid eye disease (TED), the topic of the next chapter.

CHAPTER 6

Women and Thyroid Eye Disease

This chapter is devoted to a frustrating symptom associated with thyroid disorders: thyroid eye disease, which can be disfiguring and demoralizing for women in particular. The typical scenario is to notice eye problems or changes with your eyes, only to realize there is little or no information about what's going on, what it has to do with your thyroid, what you can do to relieve your symptoms, and how you can treat the condition. And as women, we are naturally concerned with how TED affects our appearance and what we can do to downplay those effects. Unfortunately, even feminists are not immune to societal expectations about body image and appearance. Symptoms and treatment for TED are covered thoroughly, as well as self-help tips for relieving symptoms.

This chapter also explores the more general problem of dry eye syndrome, which affects roughly eleven million North Americans. So if you know someone who suffers from dry eyes, whatever the cause, be sure to pass this chapter on to her.

What Is Thyroid Eye Disease (TED)?

As if hyperthyroidism was not miserable enough, a sister disease tends to strike people with hyperthyroidism—particularly those suffering from Graves' disease and sometimes even those suffering from Hashimoto's disease. This sister disease is known as thyroid eye disease (TED). In clinical circles, TED is known by several different names:

Graves' ophthalmopathy, thyroid-associated ophthalmopathy, and, infrequently, dysthyroid orbitopathy. (The prefix "ophthalmo" means eyes, while "pathy" means disease.) It is this disease that lends itself to the expression "thyroid eyes"—bulging, watery eyes—a condition known as exophthalmos (pronounced exo-thalmus).

The most common symptom of TED is lid retraction. Here, your upper eyelids can retract slightly and expose more of the whites of your eyes. The lid retraction creates a rather dramatic "staring" look, an exaggerated expression. Sometimes the eyes improve when the hyperthyroidism is corrected. But this is not always the case, as many people with TED can attest.

When TED is associated with Graves' disease, the eye problems can be far more severe. As many as 50 percent of all Graves' disease patients suffer from TED. At one time, only those with noticeable changes to the eyes were considered to have TED, but more sophisticated methods of diagnosis reveal that eye changes are present in almost all Graves' disease patients, even though symptoms may not be noticeable. (See Figure 6.1.)

TED Alert

When you notice one or more of these seven signs of TED, request a thyroid function test. These symptoms usually appear at least a year before hyperthyroid or hypothyroid symptoms.

1. Gritty, itching, and watery eyes
2. Aching discomfort behind the eyes, especially when you look up or to the side
3. Sensitivity to light or sun
4 Congestion in the eyelids (this may be mistaken for an infection)
5. Dry eyes
6. Lid lag (where the upper lids are slow to follow when you look down)
7. Bulging eyes or a staring look (the first is caused by inflammation; the second caused by lid retraction)

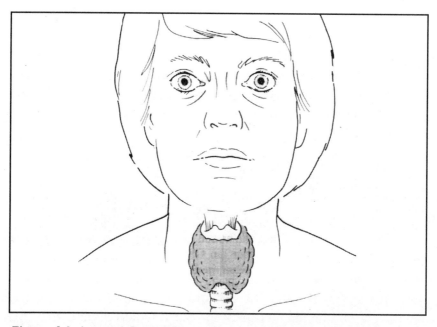

Figure 6.1 A typical Graves' disease patient with a goiter and thyroid eye
disease (TED).

Reprinted from *Nichts Gutes im Schilde Krankheiten der Schiddruse.* Copyright 1994, Georg Thieme Publishing.

The most common eye changes are bulginess and double vision
(read on). Generally, the changes to the eyes reach a "burnout" period within a two-year time frame and then stop. Sometimes the eyes
get better by themselves, but usually, after the "burnout" period, the
eyes remain changed but do not get any worse. The severity of the
eye changes can be measured by an opthalmologist (an eye disease
specialist) with an instrument called an "exophthalmometer." This
instrument measures the degree to which the eyes have become
bulgy.

The Stages of TED

In 80 percent of cases of Graves-associated TED, symptoms of TED
appear about a year before the symptoms of Graves' disease. This, of
course, can be very frustrating, and may throw your doctor off the
scent of thyroid disease altogether. See the sidebar on page 132 for
the early symptoms of TED and request a thyroid function test if you

suffer from symptoms. When symptoms first appear, TED is said to be in its active, or initial, phase. This can last anywhere from eighteen to twenty-four months. During the active phase, you will experience the most dramatic eye changes, and it is unwise to attempt to treat the condition beyond symptom relief until the eyes reach their "burnout" phase. This means the eye problem will reach a "maximum change" point, where they will probably remain changed but not worsen.

What Causes TED?

TED continues to baffle thyroid specialists and researchers. Right now, it is believed that TED is a separate disease that is aggravated by the autoimmune antibodies that develop in Graves' disease. If you had a rash caused by a food allergy, for example, and then went out in the sun, the rash would get worse rather than better. In this case, TED is the "rash" while Graves' disease is the "sun." For some strange reason, the same proteins in your thyroid cells and your eye muscle cells react to antithyroid antibodies that occur with Graves' disease. This is known as cross-reactivity. What is most baffling is why, when Graves' disease is treated, the eyes do not get better. This continues to frustrate TED sufferers.

The fact that TED can occur in the absence of Graves' disease is what makes researchers believe the two diseases are separate. There are no answers in genetic research, either; no gene has yet been found that makes one person more vulnerable to TED than another. Environment and lifestyle seem to affect TED, however. Smokers are far more likely to suffer from severe TED than nonsmokers, while stress seems to aggravate the condition, too. (In general, though, people who smoke tend to be under more stress than people who do not.)

What causes the bulging? Our eyeballs are encased in pear-shaped sockets known as orbits. The orbits of the eye are lined with pads of protective fat, connective tissue, blood vessels, muscles, nerves, and the lacrimal glands that are responsible for making tears. When the muscles that move the eyes enlarge and the fatty connective tissue

within the orbits become inflamed, the eyeballs bulge forward, causing the classic bulging eyes for which TED is infamous.

Who gets TED? You are more likely to suffer from TED if you are:
- Diagnosed with Graves' disease (see chapter 8);
- Middle-aged;
- Under stress or work in a stressful environment (see chapter 8);
- Smoke (read on).

Smoking and TED The link between smoking and TED is so strong
that thyroid specialists believe smokers with Graves' disease can probably count on developing TED. Not only is TED much less common
in nonsmokers, but some sources say it is "rare" in nonsmokers. No
one knows exactly why smokers are vulnerable to TED. What we do
know is that smokers are vulnerable to many more diseases and health
problems than nonsmokers. Clearly, TED is one of them. However,
it is certainly not surprising that an environment where you're sur-
rounded by your own (or others') cigarette smoke would aggravate—
or even help trigger—TED.

In fact, one of the reasons that nonsmokers are so uncomfortable
in smoke-filled rooms is because the smoke irritates their eyes, causing them to be watery, itchy, and red! Quitting smoking may help to
ease some of the symptoms of TED.

True Grit: The Symptoms of TED

Typical TED symptoms are caused by inflammation of the eye tissues:
the eyes become painful, red, and watery with a "gritty" feeling.
Sensitivity to light, wind, or sun are also common. The grittiness and
light sensitivity occur because of lid retraction: when your eyes are
less protected by the eyelids from dust, wind, and infection, you really feel it.

Other symptoms include discomfort when looking up or to the
side. And while some Graves' disease patients suffer from excessive
watering of the eyes, many will also suffer from excessive dryness (see
page 140). In rare and extreme cases, vision deteriorates as a result of
too much pressure being placed on the optic nerve.

The covering of the eye is also inflamed and swollen. The lids and tissues around the eyes are swollen with fluid, and the eyeballs tend to bulge out of their sockets. Because of eye muscle damage, the eyes cannot move normally, resulting in blurred or double vision.

During what's called the "hot phase," or initial active phase TED, inflammation and swelling around and behind the eye are common. This phase lasts about six months, followed by the "cold phase" where the inflammation subsides and you then notice more of the visual changes.

In severe cases, swelling may be so bad that you will find it difficult to move your eye, and you will even develop ulcers on the cornea. In most cases, both eyes are affected, but one may be worse than the other. You may also experience a phenomenon called "lid lag," when your upper lids are slow to move when you're looking down.

What you see in the mirror Not all of the symptoms of TED are visible in the mirror, but some of them are. Your eyes may look puffy, have bags under them, and look bloodshot at the corners. People may wonder why you seem to look "stunned" or amazed all the time. This will be due to your lids being retracted, thus giving you a more "dramatic" appearance. You may also be able to observe that the whites of your eyes are visible between the iris and lower lid and/or above the iris and upper lid.

Getting a Diagnosis

TED is frequently misdiagnosed as an allergy or pink eye (a.k.a. conjunctivitis). One easy way to confirm TED is to request that your thyroid be checked and also to request a thyroid antibody test. If you have noticed vision problems, you should also request screening for Type 2 diabetes. Diabetes-related eye disease is also a common problem for women over age forty-five, in particular. Imaging tests such as CT (computerized tomography), ultrasound, or MRI (magnetic resonance imaging) may be used to view the orbit or eye tissues.

Interestingly, some people will notice that TED symptoms worsen when their thyroid hormone levels are lower than normal. Because hypothyroidism causes bloating and fluid retention, this can exacerbate inflammation of the eyes, triggering TED symptoms of dryness and grit. Many thyroid patients have ongoing disputes with their physicians over whether their TED flare-up is related to their thyroid condition. It is. And since little is known about the relationship between TED and thyroid disease in general, you do not have to accept your doctor's words upon being informed that you are imagining the connection.

Battling the Bulge: Treating TED

Before specific treatments for TED begin, the thyroid condition is treated first. In some cases, when the hyperthyroidism is treated, the eyes tend to get better—even before "burnout" occurs. For example, TED in the absence of Graves' disease tends to be much easier to treat. In this case, you will probably suffer from lid retraction and some wateriness. Discomfort, redness, and intolerance of light can also be present. But when your thyroid problem is treated, your symptoms will probably disappear. This is not usually the case when TED is diagnosed alongside Graves' disease, unfortunately.

Drug Treatments

Often the first step in treating TED is to offer a steroid drug, known as prednisone, which will reduce the swelling and inflammation causing the more severe TED symptoms. Steroids have numerous side effects, however, and you'll need to balance the side effects against TED symptoms. The other problem with steroids is that once you go off of them, TED symptoms can resume, and may even get worse.

Side effects of prednisone When you're on this drug, you'll have a lower resistance to infections and may develop harder-to-treat infections. It is also associated with mood changes and insomnia that can exacerbate symptoms of thyroid disease (see chapters 2 and 3). There is a long list of other less common side effects associated with this drug, which you'll need to discuss with your doctor prior to consenting to this treatment. If you're pregnant, breast-feeding, or planning to get pregnant, you must not be on this drug, period.

Diuretics Many doctors will prescribe diuretics that cause you to urinate more frequently, thereby eliminating excess fluid. This can sometimes help to reduce swelling. Unfortunately, women at risk for osteoporosis will want to be careful that they do not eliminate calcium in their urine and will need to "top up" calcium intake while on diuretics.

Radiation

If you choose not to go on steroids, cobalt radiation therapy, or X-ray therapy, is another option. This procedure consists of X-ray, CT scans, and a simulation procedure in which careful measurements are taken in order to aim the X-ray properly; the X-ray is targeted at the muscles at the back of the eyes behind the lens—which will conceivably kill the cells causing the eye inflammation. The measurement is done using three laser light beams. About 80 percent of these treatments are successful, and the X-ray treatment is not considered harmful. This treatment usually helps to restore lost vision.

Corrective Surgery

A procedure known as orbital decompression can remove bone and expand the area behind the eye so that swollen tissue can move into it. It's best to wait until the "burnout" period before attempting surgery so the eyes do not get any worse.

There are other plastic surgery procedures that can help to reconstruct the eye area and correct the disfigurement. Before you undergo corrective surgery, it's best to consult with a surgeon who specializes in orbital surgery, facial surgery, and neurosurgery (you may need to see three different surgeons). An ear, nose, and throat specialist may also need to be consulted.

Generally, depending on your symptoms, surgery for TED can involve any of the following:

- adjusting the position of your eyelids
- correcting swelling around the eye
- realigning eye muscles
- orbital decompression

Finding Symptom Relief

To relieve irritation and inflammation, eye drops or "artificial tears" are recommended, but it's important to ask your doctor for an appropriate brand. (See page 142.) Double vision can be remedied by wearing plastic prism lenses that can be inserted inside your regular glasses, or operations that use similar techniques that correct squinting in childhood can be done at a later stage. Injecting botulinum (a food poisoning toxin that paralyzes the nerves that control the muscles) can also help correct double vision.

The following self-help tips have been compiled from TED sufferers:

- Stop smoking and/or avoid secondhand smoke
- Use artificial tears to help moisten the eyes (see the section about eye drops on page 142)
- Sleep with the head of your bed raised (put some books under the legs) or prop yourself up on pillows to drain away excess fluid and reduce puffiness and swelling around the eyes
- Cover your eyes when you sleep
- Wear wraparound dark glasses outdoors during the day
- Turn ceiling fans off before you go to bed
- Avoid strong sunlight
- Do not wear contact lenses
- Try to help relieve swelling or drink more fluids
- Use cooling eye masks and gels
- Wear a patch over one eye to help with double vision

See the next section on dry eyes (page 140) for more useful self-help tips.

Appearance Matters

Women suffering from TED may also suffer from body image problems as a result of the disfiguring symptoms. This is not unlike what cancer patients who lose their hair go through. When a disease has affected your appearance, there may be some benefit from counseling. Some of you may also benefit from a session with a professional makeup artist. To find one in your area, contact your local television station and ask who does the makeup for the newscasters. Most makeup artists work freelance and can be available to come to your home.

Book time with a makeup artist to come to your home and show you brands of hypoallergenic eye makeups that do not contain perfume. Perfumes used on other parts of the face or in your hair may also irritate your eyes, so it's best to look into it beforehand.

A good makeup artist will show you techniques to downplay the eyes or to create the impression of less swelling with good brushes and shadows. But until you can see one, you would be well advised to stop wearing eye makeup—mainly because what you are using may be harmful.

In the meantime, what you can do on your own is to accentuate your lips (there are tricks for this, too, which a good makeup artist can show you) and get a *good* haircut. Highlights or color may also work to downplay the eyes. Having your eyebrows professionally shaped so that they are even can also do wonders. Wearing fashionable, wraparound sunglasses will enable you to attend outdoor events and activities. You can also pick up fashionable clear frames that will downplay the eyes as well. Scarves and necklaces will detract attention away from the eyes, too.

Drying Your Eyes Out

Some symptoms of TED are not unique to women suffering from thyroid disease. Dry eyes are so common that a new syndrome has emerged in general medical practice, known as dry eye syndrome. It's estimated that roughly eleven million North Americans suffer from dry eyes, meaning that tear production is inadequate or the tears evaporate so quickly that your eyes are left gritty and irritated with every blink.

What is unique about dry eyes these days is that it is now observed in much younger people. In the past, dry eyes were observed in people over age sixty-five; today it is common in thirty-year-olds.

Common causes of dry eyes (which could aggravate TED) include:

- waking up (tear production decreases when we sleep, nor do we blink during sleep, which normally spreads tears over the surface of the eyes)
- wind, sun, and pollution
- smoke
- airplanes
- hotels (with "canned air")
- overly dry places or air-conditioning
- chlorine from pools
- salt water from oceans
- cycling without goggles
- contact lenses
- side effects to medications

Dry eyes can also result from focusing too long on display screens such as television or computer screens, which is one reason why experts think it's becoming increasingly common in young people.

Easy-fix solutions include using humidifiers at night and humidifying the air in winter (when furnaces can dry out the air). If your dryness is related to medication that you are taking, switching to a different brand can sometimes solve the problem, too.

Wetting Your "Windows"

If the eyes are the "windows to the soul," here are some ways to keep those windows moist:

- Hold a warm, wet washcloth over your closed lids for five to ten minutes several times a day to unclog oil glands around the eyes
- When you're involved in an outdoor sport, choose protective eyewear to preserve moisture and shield you from the wind
- Always point air vents away from your eyes—especially in cars
- When you're working on the computer or watching television, don't forget to blink
- Avoid prolonged use of hair dryers

The Trouble with Eye Drops

Using the wrong eye drops can aggravate, rather than relieve, dry eyes because they can contain irritating preservatives. Even antibiotic or antiallergenic drops can cause problems. The best solution (pardon the pun) is to ask your eye doctor to recommend something rather than an over-the-counter product.

In severe cases, you can have silicone plugs surgically inserted into the drainage ducts leading out of the eyes, which will help you retain artificial tears or jellies. This will reduce the number of times you need to use eye drops.

A woman's tears Dry eyes are considered to be a woman's problem since so many autoimmune diseases, which plague women in particular, are associated with dry eyes. Aside from Graves' disease, other autoimmune diseases causing dry eyes include Sjogren's syndrome (this impairs lacrimal gland function and the formation of watery tears; 90 percent of Sjogren's syndrome sufferers are women), rheumatoid arthritis, lupus, diabetes, and Crohn's disease.

Hormonal changes during preganncy and menopause can also cause dry eyes, while asthma, glaucoma, blepharitis (chronic inflammation of the eyelids), cornea surgery, and corrective surgery for nearsightedness are other causes.

Women are also more likely to develop dry eyes because of side effects to medications. These include antidepressants (women tend to suffer from depression more frequently than men—see chapter 3), decongestants, antihistamines, blood pressure drugs, hormones, oral contraceptives, diuretics, ulcer medications, tranquilizers, and beta-blockers.

Aging, traditionally the reason why dry eyes were most often observed in older women, is also a cause. As we age, there is a decrease in tear production in both men and women.

꙳

While TED is a symptom most often associated with hyperthyroidism and Graves' disease, weight gain is more often associated with hypothyroidism. The next chapter discusses another kind of "battle of the bulge" common to thyroid sufferers and suggests ways to win the war.

CHAPTER 7

The Weight and Diet Connection

When women think "thyroid problem," they usually think "weight problem." Weight is a complex topic for women that has as much to do with our social conditioning about body size, and what we perceive to be an acceptable weight, than it does with actual calorie intake. This chapter discusses how your thyroid problem can affect your weight and how it can aggravate a *preexisting* weight problem, which is usually the more serious consequence of a thyroid condition for most women. You will also find important fat-cutting information, as well as a discussion on "iodine foods" and how they affect a healthy thyroid gland.

Thyroid Disease and Obesity

If you weigh 20 percent more than your ideal weight for your height and age, you are technically considered obese. When obesity is due to hypothyroidism, most women will find that they return to their normal weight once their hypothyroidism is treated. Nevertheless, many women who are overweight may indeed be suffering from an undiagnosed thyroid problem. Therefore, if you are reading this chapter and wondering whether your weight problem is caused by an underactive thyroid problem or "metabolism," a simple blood test that measures your levels of thyroid-stimulating hormone will confirm whether your thyroid levels are normal. (See chapter 10.)

Feeling tired and low in energy, a symptom of hypothyroidism, can cause you to crave carbohydrates and quick-energy foods, which are higher in fat and calories. When you are hypothyroid, your activity levels will decrease as a result of your fatigue, which can also lead to weight gain. The craving for carbohydrates is caused by a desire for energy. Consuming carbohydrates produces an initial "rush" of energy, but then it is followed by a tremendous "crash," which is sometimes known as postprandial depression (or postmeal depression), exacerbating or contributing to hypothyroid-induced depression. Even in women with normal thyroid function, depression can cause cravings for simple carbohydrates such as sugars and sweets. Many women will notice that they are not craving food at all but are still gaining weight. Some of the weight gain is bloating from constipation. Increasing fluid intake and fiber will help the problem.

Obviously, cutting down on fat (see page 155) will also help. But the problem for most women who are battling both obesity and hypothyroidism is that the weight problem often predates the thyroid problem, indicating that there are other factors involved in their weight gain. Stack a thyroid problem on top of that, and it may exacerbate all kinds of other behaviors that led to the initial weight gain, as well as aggravate risks associated with obesity in general, such as Type 2 diabetes, heart disease, or stroke. This section therefore examines other factors that lead to obesity so that you can "weed out" nonthyroid and thyroid-related reasons for your weight gain.

Chronic Dieting

Many obese women say that they have "dieted themselves up" to their present weight. Indeed, the road to obesity is paved with chronic dieting. It is estimated that at least 50 percent of all North American women are dieting at any given time, while one-third of North American dieters initiate a diet at least once a month. The very act of dieting in your teens and twenties can predispose you to obesity in your thirties, forties, and beyond. This occurs because most people "crash and burn" instead of eating sensibly. In other words, they are chronic dieters.

The crash-and-burn approach to diet is what we do when we want to lose a specific number of pounds for a particular occasion or item of clothing. The pattern is to starve for a few days and then eat

Seven Tips for Active Living

If you're battling hypothyroidism, in particular, and are concerned about weight gain, it's important to remain active. This doesn't mean that you have to join a fitness club or do aerobics everyday; it simply means that you should try to incorporate some activity into your day so that you are not sedentary. Sedentary living breeds weight gain and fatigue. Here are seven tips for active living—one tip for each day of the week:

- If you drive everywhere, pick the parking space farther away from your destination in order to incorporate some daily walking into your life.
- If you take public transit everywhere, get off one or two stops early so that you can walk the rest of the way to your destination.
- Choose stairs more often rather than escalators or elevators.
- Park at one side of the mall and then walk to the opposite side.
- Take a stroll after dinner around your neighborhood.
- Volunteer to walk the dog (or somebody's dog if you do not have one).
- On weekends, go to the zoo or get out to flea markets, garage sales, and so on.

what we normally do. Or, we eat only certain foods (like celery and grapefruit) for a number of days and then eat normally after we've lost the weight. Most of these diets do not incorporate exercise, which means that we burn up some of our muscle as well as fat. Then, when we eat normally, we gain only fat. And over the years that fat simply grows fatter. The bottom line is that when there is more fat on your body than muscle, you cannot burn calories as efficiently. It is the muscle that makes it possible to burn calories. Diet it away, and you diet away your ability to burn fat.

If starvation is involved in trying to lose weight, our bodies will simply become more efficient at getting fat. Starvation triggers an intelligence in the metabolism; our body suddenly thinks we are living in a war zone and goes into "super-efficient nomadic mode." So when we return to our normal caloric intake, or even a lower-than-normal caloric intake after we've starved ourselves, *we gain more weight*. Our bodies say: "Oh look—food! Better store that as fat for the next famine." Some researchers believe that starvation diets slow down our metabolic rates far below normal so that weight gain becomes more rapid after each starvation episode.

This cycle of crash or starvation dieting is known as the yo-yo diet syndrome, the subject of thousands of articles in women's magazines throughout the last twenty years. Breaking the pattern seems easy: combine exercise with a sensible diet. But it's not that easy if you've led a sedentary life for most of your adult years. Ninety-five percent of the people who go on a diet gain back the weight they lost, as well as extra weight, within two years. As discussed further on, the failure often lies in psychological and behavioral factors. We have to understand why we need to eat before we can eat less. The best way to break the yo-yo diet pattern is to educate your children early about food habits and appropriate body weight. Experts say that unless you are significantly overweight to begin with or have a medical condition, don't diet. Just eat well.

But if you're going to diet A recent study suggests that prepackaged balanced meals can help you stick to a meal plan more easily if you do indeed need to lose weight. Therefore, plan your meals in advance with a nutritionist and try to prefreeze or refrigerate them. This will help curb impulse eating. If you are contemplating a diet, you should also consider the following:

- What is a reasonable weight, given your genetic makeup, family history, age, and cultural background? A smaller weight loss in some people can produce dramatic effects.
- Aim to lose weight at a slower rate. Too much too fast will probably lead to gaining it all back.
- Incorporate exercise into your routine, particularly activities that build muscle mass.
- Take your vitamins. Make sure you are meeting the U.S. Recommended Dietary Allowance (RDA). Many of the popular North American diets of the 1980s, for example, were nutritionally inadequate (the Beverly Hills Diet contained 0 percent of the U.S. recommendation for vitamin B_{12}).

Eating Disorders

The two most common eating disorders involve starvation. They are *anorexia nervosa* ("loss of appetite due to mental disorder") and bingeing followed by purging, known as *bulimia nervosa* ("hunger like an ox due to mental disorder"). Women will purge after a bingeing episode by inducing vomiting, abusing laxatives, diuretics, and thyroid hormone. The most horrifying examples occur in women with normal thyroid function who take thyroid hormone to deliberately speed up their metabolism. Eating disorders are diseases of control that primarily affect women, although more men have become vulnerable, too, in recent years. Bulimics and anorexics are usually overachievers in other aspects of their lives and view excess weight as an announcement to the world that they are "out of control." This view becomes more distorted as time goes on, until the act of eating food in public (for bulimics) or at all (for anorexics) is equivalent to a loss of control.

In anorexia, the person's emotional and sensual desires are perceived through food. These unmet desires are so great that the anorexic fears that once she eats she'll never stop since her appetite will know no natural boundaries. The fear of food drives the disease.

Most of us find it easier to relate to the bulimic than the anorexic; bulimics express their loss of control through bingeing in the same way that someone else may yell at his or her children. Bulimics then purge to regain their control. There is a feeling of comfort for bulimics in both the binge and the purge. Bulimics are sometimes referred to as "failed anorexics" because they would starve if they could. Anorexics, however, are masters of control. They never break. I once asked a recovering anorexic the dumb question, "But didn't you get hungry?" Her response was that the hunger pangs made her feel powerful. The more intense the hunger, the more powerful she felt; the power actually gave her a "high."

Psychological Roles of Fat

There is another part of the "weight" story that has do with the role of food and fat in women's lives. Being fat—and/or the overeating behavior that causes us to be fat—is perceived by many as a very public rebellion against the role many women are asked to play in this society. So it's important to explore what being fat means to you, personally, and the issues surrounding food addiction.

As women, we are the ones that usually do the purchasing and preparing of food for our families. But at the same time, we are continuously being deluged with impossible standards of beauty, fitness, and thinness through media images. How do these conflicting roles affect us? For many women, the effect is a feeling of powerlessness. And, depending on the woman, by manipulating one's body size to be bigger or smaller by eating food or refusing food, we express unconscious desires to achieve more control over our lives. For the record, compulsive eating is more often a woman's problem, which tells us that it has much more to do with "being a woman" than we are generally told by doctors and dietitians. Psychotherapists who specialize in compulsive eating disorders stress that the only way to help women lose weight is to help them understand what conscious or unconscious needs are being met by the fat.

The meaning of your fat Therapists who work with women about weight loss issues often observe that fat both isolates a woman on the one hand, and makes her an object of failure on the other. Women, of course, know this, and sometimes use this for psychological advantage. In other words, to the woman, the fat can "protect" her from being successful in two specific areas: sexual and financial (i.e., career-related success). Many women who are striving for financial success find that a thin body size immediately interferes with that goal. When they are thin, they fear being perceived on sexual terms by male colleagues (or have been so perceived/noticed in the past). They may even fear their own sexual desires or fear being rejected as a sexual object. But when they are fat, they can feel liberated from being perceived as a sexual or "decorative" object and enjoy the financial rewards of their success nonetheless—or simply enjoy being perceived as productive or competent.

On the flip side, many women who have never had success in their lives (sexual or financial) use their fat as a way to remain isolated. This allows them to say to themselves, "If I were thin, I'd be successful." Their fatness can become the reason for failed attempts at personal success, which can shield many women from facing their own inner demons and fears and can keep them from the success they really want.

When fat means "mother" For many women—especially women who have gained their weight after childbirth—fat has nothing to do with sexuality or personal/financial success. It has to do with their relationship with their mother and their own feelings of nurturing and being a mother. After all, it is a mother's breasts that initially nurture us, and it is through our mother that we learn about food, food behaviors, and so on. Our mothers are also the source of love, comfort, and emotional support. Even if we did not get this from our own mother, we still associate "mothering" with these emotions. Therapists have observed that body size and eating get tangled up in mother-daughter relationships and can have varied meanings for the overweight woman. In other words, what your fat says to your mother can mean anything from "I'm a big girl and can look after myself" to "I'm a mess and *can't* look after myself." Some daughters use fat to actually reject their mother's role or to express anger at their mother for inadequate nurturing.

When fat means "I'm angry" Many women find that their fat expresses a welcome anger at the beauty standard and repressive sexual role they're asked to play. The fat is not "protection," but a deliberate attempt to offend the world. Here, the fat says to the world, "If you really want to get to know me, then you'll take the time to penetrate my layers. Otherwise, I don't want to know you!"

The fear that less is more Many women fear being "seen." The belief that "the less of me there is, the more people will see" is the reason behind their fat. The fat thus protects the woman from being "overexposed" both emotionally and sexually.

Compulsive Eating

The physical symptoms associated with hypothyroidism can exacerbate the compulsive eating behavior that predates hypothyroidism. The craving for carbohydrates (see page 143) can also wreak havoc on preexisting eating behaviors. When we hear "eating disorder," we usually think about anorexia or bulimia. There are many people, however, who binge without purging. This is also known as binge eating disorder (a.k.a., compulsive overeating). In this case, bingeing is still an announcement to the world that "I'm out of control." Someone who purges is trying to hide his/her lack of control. Someone who binges and never purges is *advertising* his/her lack of control. The purger is passively asking for help; the binger who does not purge is aggressively asking for help. It's the same disease with a different result. But there is one more layer when it comes to compulsive overeating, which is considered to be controversial, and is often rejected by the overeater: a desire to get fat is often behind the compulsion. Many people who overeat insist that fat is a consequence of eating food, not a *goal*. Many therapists who deal with overeating disagree, and believe that if a woman admits that she has an emotional interest in actually being large, she may actually be much closer to stopping her compulsion to eat.

Furthermore, many women who eat compulsively do not recognize that they are doing so. The following is a typical profile of a compulsive eater:

- Eating when you are not hungry
- Feeling out of control when you are around food, either trying to resist it or gorging on it
- Spending a lot of time thinking/worrying about food and your weight
- Always desperate to try another diet that promises results
- Feelings of self-loathing and shame
- Hating your own body
- Obsessed with what you can or will eat, or have eaten
- Eating in secret or with "eating friends"
- Appearing in public to be a professional dieter who is in control
- Buying cakes or pies as "gifts" and having them wrapped to hide the fact that they are for you
- Having a "pristine" kitchen with only the "right" foods
- Feeling either out of control with food (compulsive eating) or imprisoned by it (dieting)

- Feeling temporary relief by "not eating"
- Looking forward with pleasure and anticipation to the time when you can eat alone
- Feeling unhappy because of your eating behavior

Biological Causes of Obesity

Eating too much high-fat or high-calorie food while remaining sedentary is certainly one biological cause of obesity. Furthermore, a woman's metabolism slows down by 25 percent after menopause, which means that unless she either decreases her calories by 25 percent or increases her activity level by 25 percent to compensate, she will probably gain weight. Hypothyroidism is also common in women over age fifty, which can add fuel to the fire.

Because diet and lifestyle changes are so difficult, there is an interest in finding genetic causes for obesity. That would mean that obesity is beyond our control—and something we have inherited, which would probably be comforting for many people. Now that we are in the midst of the Human Genome Project, a project that intends to map every gene in the human body, efforts are under way to find the "obesity gene" or "fat gene." But few scientists believe that obesity is *simply* genetic. In other words, there are so many environmental and societal factors that can "trip" the obesity "switch"; finding a specific gene for obesity is about as worthwhile as finding the "anger gene" or "crime gene."

Some theories An important theory about why we get fat involves insulin resistance. It's believed that when the body produces too much insulin, we will eat more to try to maintain a proper balance. This is why weight gain is often the first symptom of Type 2 diabetes. But then we have to ask what causes insulin resistance to begin with, and many researchers believe that it is triggered by obesity. So it becomes a "chicken or egg" puzzle. There are also many theories surrounding the function of fat cells. Are some people genetically programmed to have more, or "fatter," fat cells than others? There are no answers yet.

What about the brain and obesity? Some propose that obesity is "all in the head" and has something to do with the hypothalamus (a part of the brain that controls messages to other parts of the body) somehow malfunctioning when it comes to sending the body the message "I'm full." It's believed that the hypothalamus may control "satiation messages."

To other researchers, the problem has to do with some sort of "defect" in the body that does not recognize hunger cues or satiation cues, but the studies in this area are not conclusive.

What about the fat hormone? A study reported in a 1997 issue of *Nature Medicine* showed that people with low levels of the hormone leptin may be prone to weight gain. In this study, people who gained an average of fifty pounds over three years started out with lower leptin levels than people who maintained their weight over the same period. Therefore, this study may form the basis for treating obesity with leptin. Experts speculate that 10 percent of all obesity may be due to a leptin resistance. Leptin is made by fat cells and apparently sends messages to the brain about how much fat our bodies are carrying. As with other hormones, it's thought that leptin has a stimulating action that acts as a thermostat of sorts. In mice, adequate amounts of leptin somehow signaled the mouse to become more active and eat less, while too little leptin signaled the mouse to eat more while becoming less active.

Interestingly, Pima Indians who are prone to obesity were shown from blood analyses to have roughly one-third less leptin. Human studies of injecting leptin to treat obesity are in progress but to date have not proven effective.

Obesity Drugs

One of the oldest and frequently misused weight loss drugs around is, in fact, thyroid hormone. And as discussed in chapters 1 and 2, hyperthyroidism causes weight loss combined with an increase in appetite due to the body speeding up.

Until at least 1980, many women battling a weight problem were prescribed thyroid hormone by some doctors. When this practice was banned, anecdotal evidence showed that women with legitimate thyroid disorders were giving their pills to friends or family members who wanted them for weight control. Taking thyroid hormone when someone has a normal functioning thyroid will cause them to become hyperthyroid. This can have serious consequences for your heart (see chapter 2) if hyperthyroidism is prolonged.

In the not too distant past, amphetamines, or "speed," were often widely peddled to women as well by doctors, but these, too, are dangerous and can put your health at risk.

Anti-obesity pills   The U.S. government recently approved an anti-obesity pill that blocks absorption of almost one-third of the fat that people eat. One of the side effects of this new prescription drug, called orlistat (Xenical®), causes rather embarrassing diarrhea each time you eat fatty foods. To avoid the drug's side effects, simply avoid fat! The pill will also decrease absorption of vitamin D and other important nutrients—another point of caution.

Not yet available in Canada, orlistat is the first drug to fight obesity through the intestine instead of the brain. Taken with each meal, it binds to certain pancreatic enzymes to block digestion of 30 percent of the fat you ingest. How it affects the pancreas long term is not known. Combined with a sensible diet, people on orlistat lost more weight than those who didn't take it. This drug is not intended for people who need to lose a few pounds; it is designed for medically obese people. (Orlistat was also found to lower cholesterol, blood pressure, and blood sugar levels.)

One of the most controversial anti-obesity therapies was the use of fenfluramine and phentermine (Fen/Phen). Both drugs were approved for use individually more than twenty years ago, but since 1992, doctors tended to prescribe them together for long-term management of obesity. In 1996, U.S. doctors wrote a total of eighteen million monthly prescriptions for Fen/Phen. And many prescriptions were issued to people who were not obese. This is known as "off-label" prescribing. In July 1997, the U.S. Food and Drug Administration (FDA), along with researchers at the Mayo Clinic and the Mayo Foundation, issued a joint announcement warning doctors that Fen/Phen can cause heart disease. On September 15, 1997, "Fen" was taken off the market. The Fen/Phen lesson: diet and lifestyle modification are still the best pathways to wellness. (More bad news has surfaced about Fen/Phen wreaking havoc on serotonin levels, which only reinforces the Fen/Phen lesson.)

A Fen/Phen "replacement" drug, sibutramine (Meridia®) was approved in November 1997 by the FDA and is still pending approval in Canada as of this writing. Sibutramine was first developed in the late 1980s as an antidepressant but, like Fen/Phen, controls appetite through the brain's interpretation of "feeling full." Sibutramine differs from Fen/Phen in that it does not interfere with the heart.

Smoking and obesity Obviously, no health-care provider will "prescribe" nicotine or smoking to you as a "weight loss" drug, but many women will take up the habit anyway as a tool to weight loss or, worse, revisit the habit long after they have quit.

Smoking satisfies "mouth hunger"—the need to have something in your mouth. It also causes withdrawal symptoms that can drive people to eat. The best way to combat this problem is to ask your health-care team for some information on credible smoking cessation programs. There are, unfortunately, no easy answers to the dilemma of weight loss versus quitting smoking. Most health-care providers will assess your current risk of heart disease and/or stroke and help you prioritize your lifestyle changes. If you suffer from Graves' disease, smoking will also aggravate, or put you at increased risk for, thyroid eye disease (see chapter 6).

If You Are Hyperthyroid . . .

Most women concerned about "thyroid and weight" will be suffering from *hypo*thyroidism, which may have resulted from treatment for *hyper*thyroidism. If you are currently in the throes of hyperthyroidism, it's important to note that your thyroid helps to control food absorption, gastric emptying, secretion of digestive juices, and motility of the digestive tract. When you're hyperthyroid, despite a voracious appetite, you might lose weight, have diarrhea, develop mild anemia, and suffer bone loss as calcium is taken out of the blood and excreted in the urine. The calcium loss can exacerbate risk factors for osteoporosis (see chapter 5). Generally, premenopausal women need 1,000 mg of calcium per day, while a postmenopausal woman needs 1,200 to 1,500 mg of calcium daily. But you *can* help ease the unpleasantness by choosing what you eat. Increase your calcium intake by having more butter, cream, cheese, and other dairy products. This will also help to keep your weight up. Peanut butter, mayonnaise, and animal fat can help as well. To reduce diarrhea, cut down on fruit juices and fresh fruits. Peanut butter is also good for binding. Sometimes, hyperthyroid people will develop sudden lactose intolerance. This can lead to gas and other unpleasantries. Eliminate all milk products in this case, and take a calcium supplement while getting your fat from the other foods mentioned above.

Stay away from caffeine, alcohol, and cigarettes; all may stimulate your heart. You may want to take vitamin supplements as well. (Vitamins A, D, and E are stored in body fat and can be lost through excretion if you are hyperthyroid.) When you are in balance again, you will need to cut down on your fat and calcium intake.

Making Changes and Cutting Fat

Variety is the key to a healthy diet. If your meal contains mostly carbohydrates (50 to 55 percent), some protein (15 to 20 percent), not much fat (less than 30 percent), and limited sugar, then you are eating well.

Imagine yourself in a supermarket with a shopping cart. What you need to live is usually found on the outside aisles of any supermarket or grocery store. Outside aisles simulate the foods you can buy at outdoor markets: fruits, vegetables, meat, eggs, fish, breads, and dairy products. Natural fiber (both soluble and insoluble), discussed below, is also found in the outside aisles. But remember: foods you buy in the outside aisles can also be high in fat unless you choose wisely.

The inside aisles are not only the aisles of temptation, they may have complicated food labels. Since 1993, food labels have been adhering to strict guidelines set out by the FDA and U.S. Department of Agriculture's (USDA) Food Safety and Inspection Service (FSIS). All labels will list "Nutrition Facts" on the side or back of the package.

The "Percent Daily Values" column tells you how high or low that food is in various nutrients such as fat, saturated fat, and cholesterol. A number of 5 or less is "low"—good news if the product shows < 5 for fat, saturated fat, and cholesterol; bad news if the product is < 5 for fiber. Serving sizes are also confusing. Foods that are similar are given the same *type* of serving size defined by the FDA. That means that five cereals that all weigh X grams per cup will share the same serving sizes.

Calories (how much energy) and calories from fat (how much fat) are also listed per serving of food. Total carbohydrate, dietary fiber, sugars, other carbohydrates (which means starches), total fat, saturated fat, cholesterol, sodium, potassium, and vitamins and minerals are given in Percent Daily Values, based on the 2,000-calorie diet recommended by the U.S. government. (In Canada, Recommended Nutrient Intake (RNI) is used for vitamins and minerals, while ingredients on labels are listed according to weight with the "most" listed first.)

But that's not where the confusion ends—or even begins! You have to wade through the various "claims" to understand what they mean. For example, anything that is "X-free" (as in sugar-free, saturated fat-free, cholesterol-free, sodium-free, calorie-free, and so on) means that the product indeed has "no X" or that "X" is so tiny that it is dietarily insignificant. This is not the same thing as a label that says "95 percent fat-free." In the latter case, the product contains relatively small amounts of fat, but still has fat. This claim is based on 100 grams of the product. For example, if a snack food contains 2.5 g of fat per 50 g, it can be said to be "95 percent fat-free."

A label that screams "low in saturated fat" or "low in calories" is *not* fat-free or calorie-free. It means that you can eat a large amount of that food without exceeding the Daily Value for that food. In potato-chip country, that translates to mean that you can eat twelve potato chips instead of six. So if you eat the whole bag of "low-fat" chips, you are still eating a lot of fat. Be sure to check serving sizes.

"Cholesterol-free" or "low cholesterol" means that the product does not have any, or as much, animal fat (hence, cholesterol). This does not mean "low fat." Pure vegetable oil does not come from animals but is pure fat nevertheless.

"Less and more" And then there are the "comparison claims" such as "fewer," "reduced," "less," "more," or, my favorite—"light" (or worse, "lite"). These appear on foods that have been nutritionally altered from a previous "version" or competitor's version. For example, *Brand X Potato Chips–Regular* may have much more fat than *Brand X Potato Chips–Lite* ("With Less Fat than Regular Brand X"). That doesn't mean that Brand X Lite is fat-free or even low in fat. It just means that it's some percent *lower* in fat than Brand X Regular.

On the flip side, *Brand Y* may have a trace amount of calcium, while *Brand Y–"Now with More Calcium"* may still have a small amount of calcium, but 10 percent more than Brand Y. (In other words, you may still need to eat one hundred bowls of Brand Y before you get the daily requirement for calcium.)

To be light or "lite," a product has to contain either one-third fewer calories or half the fat of the regular product. Or, a low-calorie or low-fat food contains 50 percent less sodium. Something that is "light in sodium" means it has at least 50 percent less sodium than the regular product, such as canned soup.

What Is Fat?

Fat is technically known as *fatty acids,* which are crucial nutrients for our cells. We cannot live without fatty acids, or fat. Fat is therefore a good thing—in moderation. But, like all good things, most of us want too much of it. Excess dietary fat is by far the most damaging element in the Western diet. A gram of fat contains twice the amount of calories as the same amount of protein or carbohydrate. Fat in the diet comes from meats, dairy products, and vegetable oils. Other sources of fat include coconuts (60 percent), peanuts (78 percent), and avocados (82 percent). There are different kinds of fatty acids in these sources of fats: saturated, unsaturated, and trans-fatty acids (a.k.a. transfat). They are like a saturated fat in disguise. Some fats are harmful, while others are considered beneficial to your health.

Saturated fat Saturated fat is solid at room temperature and stimulates cholesterol production in your body. In fact, the way the fat looks prior to ingesting it is the way it will look when it lines your arteries.

Foods high in saturated fat include processed meat, fatty meat, lard, butter, margarine, solid vegetable shortening, chocolate, and tropical oils (coconut oil is more than 90 percent saturated). Saturated fat should be consumed only in very low amounts.

Unsaturated fat Unsaturated fat is partially solid or liquid at room temperature. This group of fats includes monounsaturated fats, poly-unsaturated fats, and omega-3 oils (a.k.a. fish oil), which, in fact, even protect you against heart disease (see below). Sources of unsaturated fats include vegetable oils (canola, safflower, sunflower, corn), seeds, and nuts. To make it easy to remember, unsaturated fats come from plants, with the exception of tropical oils, such as coconut. The more liquid the fat, the more polyunsaturated it is, which, in fact, *lowers* your cholesterol. However, if you have familial hyperlipidemia (high cholesterol), which often occurs along with diabetes, unsaturated fat may not make any difference in your cholesterol levels.

Fish fat (omega-3 oils) The fats naturally present in fish that swim in cold water, known as omega-3 fatty acids (crucial for brain tissue), or fish oils, are all polyunsaturated. They lower your cholesterol levels and protect against heart disease. These fish have a layer of fat to keep them warm in cold water. Mackerel, albacore tuna, salmon, sardines, and lake trout are all rich in omega-3 fatty acids. In fact, whale meat and seal meat, which once were staples of the Inuit diet in North America, are enormous sources of omega-3 fatty acids. Overhunting and federal moratoriums on whale and seal hunting have dried up this once-vital source of food for the Inuit. It clearly offered real protection against heart disease.

Man-made Fats

An assortment of man-made fats have been introduced into our diet, courtesy of food producers who are trying to give us the taste of fat without all the calories or harmful effects of saturated fats. Unfortunately, man-made fats offer their own bag of horrors.

Trans-fatty acids (a.k.a. hydrogenated oils) These are harmful fats that not only raise the level of "bad" cholesterol (LDL) in your bloodstream but also lower the amount of "good" cholesterol (HDL) that's already there. Trans-fatty acids are what you get when you make a liquid oil, such as corn oil, into a more solid or spreadable substance, such as margarine. Trans-fatty acids, you might say, are the "road to hell, paved with good intentions." Someone, way back when, thought that if you could take the "good fat"—unsaturated fat—and solidify it, so it could double as butter or lard, you could eat the same things without missing the spreadable fat. That seemed a great idea. Unfortunately, to make an unsaturated liquid fat increasingly solid, you have to add hydrogen to its molecules. This is known as *hydrogenation,* the process that converts liquid fat to semisolid fat. That ever-popular chocolate bar ingredient, "hydrogenated palm oil," is a classic example of a trans-fatty acid. Hydrogenation also prolongs the shelf life of a fat, such as polyunsaturated fats, which can oxidize when exposed to air, causing rancid odors or flavors. Deep-frying oils used in the restaurant trade are generally hydrogenated.

Trans-fatty acid is sold as a polyunsaturated or monounsaturated fat accompanied by a suitable language, such as "Made from polyunsaturated vegetable oil." Except that, once in your body, it is treated as a saturated fat. This is why trans-fatty acids are saturated fat in disguise. The advertiser may, in fact, say that the product contains "no saturated fat" or is "healthier" than the comparable animal or tropical oil product with saturated fat. So be careful and read your labels. The magic word you are looking for is hydrogenated. If the product lists a variety of unsaturated fats (monounsaturated X oil, polyunsaturated Y oil, and so on), keep reading. If the word *hydrogenated* appears, count that product as a saturated fat; your body will!

Margarine versus butter There's an old tongue twister: "Betty Botter bought some butter that made the batter bitter; so Betty Botter bought more butter that made the batter better." Are we making our batters bitter or better with margarine? It depends.

Since the news concerning trans-fatty acids broke in the late 1980s, margarine manufacturers began to offer less "bitter" margarines; some contain no hydrogenated oils, while others have much smaller amounts. Margarines with less than 60 to 80 percent oil (9 to 11 g of fat) will contain 1.0 to 3.0 g of trans-fatty acid per serving, compared to butter, which is 53 percent saturated fat. You might say this is a choice between a bad fat and a *worse* fat.

It's also possible for a liquid vegetable oil to retain a high concentration of unsaturated fat when it is been partially hydrogenated. In this case, your body will metabolize this as both saturated and unsaturated fat.

Fake fat We have artificial sweeteners; why not artificial fat? This question has led to the creation of an emerging yet highly suspicious ingredient: *fat substitutes,* designed to replace real fat and hence reduce the calories from real fat without compromising taste. This is done by creating a fake fat that the body cannot absorb.

One of the first fat substitutes was Simplesse®, an all-natural fat substitute made from milk and egg-white protein, which was developed by the NutraSweet Company. Simplesse apparently adds one to two calories per gram instead of the usual nine calories per gram from fat. Other fat substitutes simply take protein and carbohydrates and modify them to simulate the textures of fat (creamy, smooth, etc.). All of these fat substitutes help to create low-fat products.

The calorie-free fat substitute being promoted lately is olestra, developed by Proctor & Gamble. It is currently being test-marketed in the U.S. in a variety of savory snacks such as potato chips and crackers. Olestra is a potentially dangerous ingredient that most experts feel can do more harm than good. Canada has not yet approved it.

Olestra is made from a combination of vegetable oils and sugar. Therefore, it tastes just like the real thing, but its biochemical structure is a molecule too big for your liver to break down. So, olestra just gets passed into the large intestine and is excreted. Olestra is more than an "empty" molecule, however. It can cause diarrhea and cramps and may deplete your body of vital nutrients, including vitamins A, D, E, and K, the latter being necessary for blood to clot. If the FDA approves olestra for use as a cooking-oil substitute, you will see it in every imaginable high-fat product. The danger is that, instead of encouraging people to choose nutritious foods such as fruits, grains, and vegetables over high-fat foods, products such as these encourage a high *fake*-fat diet that's still too low in fiber and other essential nutrients. And the no-fat icing on the cake is that these people could potentially wind up with a vitamin deficiency to boot. Products like olestra should make you nervous.

Fiber

For every action, there is an equal and opposite reaction. When you decrease your fat intake, you should increase your bulk intake, or fiber. Complex carbohydrates are foods that are high in fiber. Fiber is the part of a plant your body can't digest (see Table 7.1). It comes in the form of both water-soluble fiber (which dissolves in water) and water-insoluble fiber (which does not disolve but, instead, absorbs water); this is what is meant by "soluble" and "insoluble" fiber.

Soluble Versus Insoluble Fiber

Soluble and insoluble fiber do differ, but they are equally good things. Soluble fiber—somehow—lowers the "bad" cholesterol, or LDL, in your body. Experts are not entirely sure how soluble fiber works its magic, but one popular theory is that it gets mixed into the bile the liver secretes and forms a type of gel that traps the building blocks of cholesterol, thus lowering your LDL levels. It is akin to a spiderweb trapping smaller insects. Sources of soluble fiber include oats or oat bran, legumes (dried beans and peas), some seeds, carrots, oranges, bananas, and other fruits. Soybeans are also high sources of soluble fiber. Studies show that people with very high cholesterol have the most to gain by eating soybeans. Soybean is also a phyto-estrogen (plant estrogen) that is believed to lower the risk of estrogen-related cancers (for example, breast cancer), as well as lower the incidence of estrogen-loss symptoms associated with menopause.

Insoluble fiber does not affect your cholesterol levels at all, but it does regulate your bowel movements. How does it do this? As the insoluble fiber moves through your digestive tract, it absorbs water like a sponge and helps to form your waste into a solid form faster, making the stools larger, softer, and easier to pass. Without insoluble fiber, your solid waste just gets pushed down to the colon or lower intestine as always, where it is stored and dried out until you are ready

Table 7.1 How Your Food Breaks Down

Complex Carbohydrates *(digest more slowly)*

- fruits
- vegetables (corn, potatoes, etc.)
- grains (breads, pastas, cereals)
- legumes (dried beans, peas, lentils)

Simple Carbohydrates *(digest quickly)*

- fruits/fruit juices
- sugars (sucrose, fructose, etc.)
- honey
- corn syrup
- sorghum
- date sugar
- molasses
- lactose

Proteins *(digest slowly)*

- lean meats
- fatty meats
- poultry
- fish
- eggs
- low-fat cheese
- high-fat cheese
- legumes
- grains

Fats *(digest slowly)*

- high-fat dairy products (butter or cream)
- oils (canola/corn/olive/safflower/sunflower)
- lard
- avocados
- olives
- nuts
- fatty meats

Fiber *(does not digest; goes through you)*

- whole-grain breads
- cereals (i.e., oatmeal)
- all fruits
- legumes (beans and lentils)
- leafy greens
- cruciferous vegetables

to have a bowel movement. High-starch foods are associated with drier stools. This is exacerbated when you "ignore the urge," as the colon will dehydrate the waste even more until it becomes harder and difficult to pass, a condition known as constipation. Insoluble fiber will help to regulate your bowel movements by speeding things along. It is also linked to lower rates of colorectal cancer. Good sources of insoluble fiber are wheat bran and whole grains, skins from various fruits and vegetables, seeds, leafy greens, and cruciferous vegetables (cauliflower, broccoli, brussels sprouts).

Breads

For thousands of years, cooked whole grains were the dietary staple for all cultures: rice and millet in the Orient; wheat, oats, and rye in Europe; buckwheat in Russia; sorghum in Africa; barley in the Middle East; and corn in pre-European North America.

Whole-grain breads are good sources of insoluble fiber (flax bread is particularly good because flaxseeds are a source of soluble fiber, too). The problem is in understanding what is truly a "whole grain." For example, there is an assumption that because bread is dark or brown, it's more nutritious; this isn't so. In fact, many brown breads are simply enriched white breads dyed with molasses. ("Enriched" means that nutrients lost during processing have been replaced.) High-fiber pita breads and bagels are available but you have to search for them. A good rule is to simply look for the phrase *whole wheat*, which means that the wheat is, indeed, whole.

"Iodine Foods" and the Thyroid

If you have a normal functioning thyroid gland but are concerned that you are at risk for a thyroid problem, is there a "thyroid disease prevention diet" you can follow?

Well . . . it will depend on where you live. We know, for example, that a lack of iodine can cause the thyroid gland to enlarge (see chapter 1). By the same token, too much iodine is believed to be responsible for triggering goiters and thyroid disorders, too. That's one reason why taking kelp (seaweed) is not recommended. If you live in

North America, you're getting enough iodine in your diet from your food. Taking kelp in the belief that it will prevent a thyroid problem is simply bad practice. Not only will it *not* prevent a thyroid problem, it could trigger one.

Hong Kong's Consumer Council had concerns about seaweed snacks that were popular with Hong Kong children. Apparently, the amount of iodine in two small packages of "roasted iodine" exceeded the World Health Organization's recommended daily iodine intake for children under age twelve. The council was concerned that the snacks could trigger goiters and thyroid disorders.

Sources of Iodine

In North America, other than recommending against taking kelp, physicians do not generally issue warnings to people at risk for a thyroid disorder about avoiding iodine-containing food. That's because you'll find iodine in a host of different foods that offer important nutrients. They include:

- Fish and seafood (e.g., clams, shrimp, haddock, halibut, oysters, salmon, sardines, tuna—this, along with meat sources, provides about 11 percent of our iodine)
- Meat (e.g., beef, lamb, beef liver—this, along with fish/seafood, provides about 11 percent of our iodine)
- Dairy: eggs, milk, butter, cream, cottage cheese, cheddar cheese (provides approximately 56 percent of our iodine)
- Fruits and vegetables: pineapple, spinach, lettuce, green peppers, raisins, seaweed
- Nuts and grains (e.g., peanuts, whole meal bread—this provides approximately 16 percent of our iodine)
- Sea salt or iodized salt
- Sugar (this provides about 11 percent of our iodine)
- Water (this provides about 4 percent of our iodine)

Your thyroid gland will use about a milligram of iodine per week (or 90 mcg per day) to make thyroid hormone; that is a tiny amount, so it is easy to understand that a balanced diet provides more than enough iodine for the average thyroid gland. A healthy thyroid gland can store enough iodine to last for three months. How much food do you need to eat to reach 90 mcg? Well, one small carton of yogurt contains 125 g of iodine, which is equivalent to 125,000,000 mcg. Don't let any of this scare you, though. A healthy thyroid gland is designed to take what it needs from your daily diet.

According to some sources, a diet too high in fiber may prevent your gut from absorbing *enough* iodine, however, while a strict sodium-free or salt-free diet may also prevent you from absorbing enough. Given that iodine is present in so many foods, it's unlikely that you're suffering from iodine deficiency in North America.

Goitrogens

These are chemicals that block, or interfere with, iodine absorption. Known goitrogens include vegetables from the brassica family (cabbage, turnips, kohlrabi, bean sprouts, cauliflower), almonds, sweet corn, and some dairy products (it depends on whether the suckling calf's mother was "dining" on goitrogenic veggies). But unless your diet contained *only* goitrogens (which it does not), there is no need to worry about having these foods as they are excellent sources of fiber, important vitamins, and cancer-fighting agents.

❧

One reason why watching your iodine intake isn't all that helpful in preventing thyroid disease is because the most common thyroid diseases are autoimmune diseases, which are believed to be triggered by stress. The next chapter is the one to read if you are concerned about how stress affects your thyroid gland. It also explains autoimmune disease in detail.

CHAPTER 8

The Stress Connection: Autoimmune Thyroid Disorders

Two of the most common thyroid diseases, Graves' disease and Hashimoto's disease, are autoimmune disorders, meaning that the body attacks its own tissues. Women are more prone to autoimmune disorders because of a natural immune suppression that occurs during pregnancy (see chapter 4). Autoimmune disorders are also triggered by stress. We live in stressful times where roughly 40 percent of all women are not only doing "double duty" by working and raising children but also may be caring for an ailing parent.

This chapter explains what an autoimmune disorder is and discusses Graves' disease and Hashimoto's disease in detail. It also discusses the role of stress, other common stress-related disorders in women, and suggests ways to "downshift" and cope with external stress.

What Is an Autoimmune Disorder?

The word *autoimmune* means "self-attacking." But before you can really grasp what this means, it's important to understand how your body normally fights off infection or disease.

Whenever an invading virus or cell is detected, your body produces specific "armies" called antibodies, which attack foreign intruders known as antigens. Antibodies are made from one type of white blood cell (called lymphocytes), and each antibody is designed for a specific virus in the same way that a key is designed for a specific lock. The antibody acts as the key, while the antigen, or "intruder," is the lock. For example, if you had contracted the chicken pox as a child, you cannot contract it again; your body is armed with the antibody that kills the chicken pox virus. But the specific chicken pox antibody is useless against all other viruses, such as the mumps or measles.

Often, our doctors give us vaccines to prevent the development of a particular virus, such as polio, for example. Vaccines work like this: the serum contains a small amount of a particular virus in a deadened, noncontagious form. Essentially, the vaccine shows your body a "picture" of the virus. The vaccine serum then stimulates your system to produce a specific antibody to combat the unwanted virus. Later, if you catch the virus, your body will destroy it before it can do any damage. That's why you don't necessarily need to get chicken pox to be protected from it; you can be vaccinated against it instead. However, creating a vaccine is a painstaking, complicated process, and it can take years for scientists to develop vaccines to combat specific viruses. Polio struck at epidemic proportions throughout the 1940s and 1950s until a vaccine was discovered.

With an autoimmune disorder, your body loses the ability to distinguish foreign tissue from normal tissue. It confuses the two and perceives healthy organs as invading viruses. Your body then winds up attacking its own organs. Some doctors describe it as a sort of allergy, where your body is in fact allergic to itself. So in the same way that the body develops specific antibodies to fight specific infections, in this case the body develops specific antibodies to attack specific organs. These are also known as autoantibodies. Many kinds of illnesses are in fact autoimmune disorders; Graves' disease and Hashimoto's disease are two of them.

Who Is Vulnerable?

Generally, anyone can develop an autoimmune disorder. Many auto-immune disorders are hereditary, while some disorders—although not hereditary—run strongly in families. This is referred to as a genetic tendency or inherited predisposition.

There is a great deal of evidence, though, to suggest that stress is a major factor in triggering an autoimmune disorder. When you are under unusual or extreme stress, depression or exhaustion can set in, which will weaken your immune system. What is labeled "unusual" or "extreme"? A death or a tragedy in the family is considered to be extremely stressful. Starting a new job, moving, or relocating is also very stressful; getting married or having a new baby is stressful. Generally, any major change in our daily routine—whether positive or negative—is stressful, but people cope with change differently. What one person finds stressful may not bother another person at all.

Women who are either pregnant or have just given birth, however, are particularly vulnerable to autoimmune disorders for reasons explained in chapter 4.

Autoimmune Thyroid Diseases

The most common autoimmune thyroid disease is Graves' disease. Named after Robert Graves, the nineteenth-century Irish physician who first recognized the condition, Graves' disease tends to affect younger and middle-aged women—usually between ages twenty to forty and during their childbearing years. It is also not unheard of for someone in her fifties or sixties to develop Graves' disease.

Statistically, Graves' disease occurs fifteen to twenty times more frequently in women than men. Roughly 1 percent of the population has Graves' disease, which includes former U.S. President George Bush, former First Lady Barbara Bush, and their dog. The late John F. Kennedy Jr. suffered from Graves' disease as well as Addison's disease. (Discussed later on, Addison's disease is also an autoimmune disorder; it also affected President John F. Kennedy.) At one time, the Bushes' Graves' disease was considered a mutual and medically fantastic coincidence, but some data have suggested that there may be an infectious agent at work that is associated with Graves' disease. Some investigators wonder whether German measles (rubella) may also trigger autoimmune thyroid disease. This may explain why there seem to be "families" of Graves' patients. At a 1994 Graves' disease convention I attended, one endocrinologist talked about testing the Bushes for this infectious agent (they tested positive). To date, the infection theory is still just that—a theory. Much more study is needed before there's a clear-cut answer.

Although there is strong evidence for the hereditary nature of Graves' disease, some doctors prefer to classify it as a disorder that "runs strongly in families." That's because no specific gene responsible for Graves' disease has been isolated.

What happens in Graves' disease? Here, an abnormal antibody is produced, called thyroid stimulating antibody (TSA). TSA stimulates the thyroid gland to vastly overproduce thyroid hormone. Normally controlled by the pituitary gland, the thyroid gets confused and is tricked into being controlled by abnormal antibodies. The result is hyperthyroidism, and a goiter almost always develops. Yet sometimes the goiter is so slight that your doctor cannot feel it.

Generally, the symptoms of Graves' disease are identical to symptoms of hyperthyroidism (see chapter 2)—a condition caused by Graves' disease.

Graves' disease and stress A recent study that surveyed Graves' patients and non-Graves' patients found that more Graves' disease patients were under stress. Experts believe that once the stressful period is over and the weakened immune system bounces back to normal function, it may bounce back too aggressively and "attack" normal tissue. It's much like a puppy that has been cooped up all day; once released from its crate, it will go crazy and jump all over you, perhaps even biting you too hard because it is not aware of its own strength.

Diagnosing and treating Graves' disease Again, the signs of Graves' disease are often obvious: you may develop a goiter and display all the classic signs of hyperthyroidism. Or you may develop thyroid eye disease symptoms, which are usually telltale signs of Graves' disease. When the signs are obvious, your doctor simply confirms the diagnosis with blood tests that check your thyroid blood levels and check for the presence of thyroid antibodies in the blood.

If you're not showing any blatant signs of hyperthyroidism but suspect Graves' disease because it runs in your family or you're experiencing more subtle symptoms, Graves' disease is again detected through blood tests that check thyroid function. If your thyroid function tests confirm hyperthyroidism, your doctor will then test for the presence of thyroid antibodies in your blood. Since Graves' disease is responsible for 80 percent of all hyperthyroid cases, most doctors routinely screen for it when hyperthyroidism is diagnosed.

There is no way to treat the root cause of Graves' disease—the autoimmune disorder itself. Therefore, treating Graves' disease involves treating the hyperthyroid symptoms. To treat hyperthyroidism, the thyroid gland is usually rendered inactive with antithyroid drugs or radioactive iodine or is removed by surgery.

To deaden the thyroid gland, radioactive iodine is the most common treatment. Radioactive iodine is simply iodine in radioactive form. Since the thyroid naturally absorbs iodine to function, when the iodine is tainted or made radioactive, the malfunctioning thyroid gland greedily absorbs it and basically destroys itself in the process. (There is usually some residual thyroid function left.) Although this seems a rather drastic and gruesome description, the procedure isn't dangerous, and there are usually no side effects other than some minor swelling or irritation to the throat. The only time radioactive iodine isn't used is when patients are under age twenty. As a precaution, children and young adults usually aren't exposed to radiation (although in over thirty-five years of active use, radioactive iodine has not yet proved harmful). Taken in either capsule form or a water-type liquid, radioactive iodine effectively destroys the thyroid gland. (See chapter 10 for a detailed discussion of radioactive iodine.) There is usually a waiting period after the radioactive iodine treatment is administered to determine if the thyroid's function has lowered. Usually the doctor will wait until you are hypothyroid before prescribing thyroid replacement hormone—to replace the output of a functioning thyroid. If your thyroid gland remains hyperthyroid after the first radioactive iodine treatment, a second dosage will be administered. Sometimes three or more doses have to be applied.

The second most common treatment is either a partial or total thyroidectomy (surgical removal of the thyroid gland). A thyroidectomy might be performed when there is either a goiter or the patient is under age twenty. This major surgery involves a general anesthetic and postsurgical stay in the hospital of at least two days. A waiting period again is involved as well. Sometimes, small pieces of thyroid tissue are left behind that could potentially reactivate Graves' disease. If this happens, radioactive iodine is used to kill off the remaining bits of tissue. When you become hypothyroid, thyroid replacement hormone will be prescribed.

Sometimes, doctors prefer to treat Graves' disease with antithyroid drugs. These drugs prevent the thyroid from manufacturing thyroid hormone. Then, as the production of hormone decreases, the hyperthyroidism will disappear. Usually, antithyroid drugs are used if patients are under age twenty, but some doctors prefer to use them at any age. Sometimes, patients themselves opt to try antithyroid drugs before more drastic measures are taken. In general, antithyroid drugs are effective about 50 percent of the time, but some doctors report just a 30 percent success rate. These low "success rates" represent remission rates rather than control rates, so interpreting antithyroid statistics correctly is important. Graves' disease, in virtually all patients, can be easily controlled with antithyroid medication. This means that the hyperthyroid symptoms caused by Graves' disease subside with antithyroid medication. However, when patients are taken off the drugs, only about 40 percent of them actually experience true remission, while the remaining 60 percent will experience a recurrence of Graves' disease. Why even bother with antithyroid medication then? Because many doctors feel that Graves' disease patients should have a chance at remission initially before more drastic therapies are used. It takes about six to eight weeks on the medication for the thyroid to resume normal function, but patients are usually kept on them for months or even years to determine if a true remission will occur. In the end, at least half the patients on antithyroid drugs wind up having either a thyroidectomy or radioactive iodine treatment. There is an upside to antithyroid drugs, however. Patients with eye problems will experience more improvement in their eyes while on antithyroid medication than with other forms of treatment.

A final note on treatment of Graves' disease: occasionally, after radioactive iodine treatment or surgery, just enough of the thyroid gland remains to function normally on its own. This means that thyroid replacement hormone is not necessary. This is not the norm, however. If you have Graves' disease, it's far more realistic to assume that after treatment you'll need to be put on thyroid replacement hormone for life. There is data that radioactive iodine therapy doesn't work as well on Graves' disease patients who were treated with antithyroid medication first. If you're having radioactive iodine therapy while still on antithyroid medication, the current literature suggests higher doses of radioactive iodine if you've been *pretreated* with antithyroid medication. The general recommendation is to avoid antithyroid medication if a doctor knows for certain that you'll be having radioactive iodine therapy.

Hashimoto's disease Not nearly as serious as Graves' disease, Hashimoto's disease is another common autoimmune disorder, also known as Hashimoto's thyroiditis. It is important to note, however, that there are other forms of thyroiditis which are not autoimmune disorders (discussed in chapter 2). In medical circles, Hashimoto's disease is referred to as chronic lymphocytic thyroiditis because of the involvement of self-attacking lymphocytes. This disease is named after Hakaru Hashimoto, the Japanese physician who first described the condition in 1912.

Like Graves' disease, Hashimoto's disease is also inherited, but most of the time Hashimoto's disease strikes women over age forty (though many younger women have also been diagnosed with it). Statistically, 1 in 10 women will likely develop Hashimoto's disease in her lifetime.

Hashimoto's disease is caused by abnormal blood antibodies and white blood cells attacking and damaging thyroid cells. Eventually, this constant attack destroys many of the thyroid cells; the absence of sufficient thyroid cells causes hypothyroidism. In most cases a goiter develops because of the inflammation, though sometimes the thyroid gland can actually shrink.

If you develop Hashimoto's disease, you probably will not notice any symptoms. Sometimes there is a mild pressure in the thyroid gland and fatigue can set in, but unless you are on the lookout for thyroid disease, Hashimoto's disease can go undetected for years. Only when the thyroid cells are damaged to the point that the thyroid gland functions inadequately will you begin to experience the symptoms of hypothyroidism, described in chapter 2.

In rare instances, thyroid eye disease can set in as well. Again, the antibodies produced in Hashimoto's disease most likely aggravate the proteins in the eye muscle. Treating eye problems associated with Hashimoto's disease involves treating the initial hypothyroidism first. If eye problems persist, the same treatment pattern outlined for Graves' disease will be necessary.

Rarer still, some people with Hashimoto's disease experience hyperthyroidism *as well as* hypothyroidism. This hyper/hypo "combination" sometimes occurs due to two antibodies at work: those that attack and destroy thyroid cells and those that stimulate the gland to overproduce thyroxine—exactly like the antibodies involved with Graves' disease. This condition is coined "Hashitoxicosis." Anyone suffering from this somewhat paradoxical condition would *first* experience all the symptoms of Graves' disease. After a few months, the antibodies attacking the thyroid cells will usually overpower the Graves'-like antibodies, and the hyperthyroidism will cure itself.

Then, as Hashimoto's disease progresses, you would eventually become hypothyroid unless a replacement hormone was prescribed.

Diagnosis and treatment of Hashimoto's disease   The signs of Hashimoto's disease are not at all obvious. In its early stages, a goiter can develop as a result of inflammation in the thyroid gland. The goiter is usually firm but in rare cases can actually be tender. The goiter's tenderness can suggest Hashimoto's disease, but it is usually suspected because of the onset of sudden hypothyroidism or the age of a hypothyroid patient, given that it is common in women over age forty. Hashimoto's disease is frequently misdiagnosed, however. Often, hypothyroidism is attributed to age—particularly in women entering menopause.

Hashimoto's disease is easily diagnosed through a blood test that indicates high levels of antibodies in the blood. Another method of confirming diagnosis is through a needle biopsy. Here, a needle is inserted into the thyroid gland to remove some cells. The cells are then smeared onto a glass slide which, in the case of Hashimoto's disease, would reveal abnormal white blood cells.

The treatment is simple: thyroid replacement hormone is prescribed as soon as the diagnosis is made—even if there are no symptoms. There are three reasons why this is done. First, the synthetic hormone suppresses production of thyroid stimulating hormone (TSH) by the pituitary gland, which, in turn, shrinks any goiter that may have developed or is about to develop. Second, because Hashimoto's disease often progresses to the point where hypothyroidism sets in, the synthetic hormone nips hypothyroidism in the bud and prevents the Hashimoto's patient from suffering the unpleasant symptoms of hypothyroidism. Finally, for some reason, synthetic thyroid hormone seems to interfere with the blood antibodies that are attacking the thyroid gland.

If you have developed a goiter as a result of Hashimoto's disease, the goiter usually persists unless thyroid hormone is prescribed. Occasionally, though, the goiter shrinks on its own. On average, it takes anywhere from six to eighteen months for the goiter to shrink, and, when it does shrink, you will most certainly be hypothyroid. However, most often a shrunken thyroid gland is small from the beginning. (Remember, a goiter is simply an enlarged thyroid gland, so when the thyroid gland shrivels up, it no longer functions.) In rare instances, goiters can persist—despite synthetic thyroxine—for years.

Other Common Autoimmune Disorders

If you have one autoimmune disease, you are more likely to start a "collection" of them. Graves' disease and Hashimoto's disease are associated with other conditions, just as Graves' disease is associated with thyroid eye disease. The most common autoimmune disorders thyroid sufferers are at risk for include the following.

Anemia When you're anemic, there's a decrease in the number of red blood cells carrying oxygen to various body tissues. Often, people who are hypothyroid are mildly anemic because of the body's tendency to slow its functions. There are usually no specific symptoms associated with mild anemia, and it corrects itself when hypothyroidism is treated. A more serious type of anemia—pernicious (meaning serious) anemia—tends to occur in older people who either have or have had Grave's disease or Hashimoto's disease. Pernicious anemia is caused by a deficiency of vitamin B_{12} (the vitamin responsible for producing red blood cells). When your thyroid is functioning normally, cells lining the stomach produce "intrinsic factor," which enables the body to absorb vitamin B_{12} from food. Self-attacking antibodies to "intrinsic factor" occur in this disorder. Thus, they can be considered an associated autoimmune disease genetically related to Graves' or Hashimoto's disease (like the eye disease). The interference can prevent the body from absorbing the vitamin B_{12} it needs to manufacture sufficient quantities of red blood cells. When vitamin B_{12} levels drop, anemia can set in.

Symptoms of pernicious anemia include numbness and tingling in the hands and feet (this happens because vitamin B_{12} also nourishes the nervous system), loss of balance, and leg weakness. Studies suggest that 5 percent of those diagnosed with Graves' disease and 10 percent of those diagnosed with Hashimoto's disease may develop pernicious anemia. However, because this type of anemia usually develops in patients over age sixty, younger patients with either Graves' or Hashimoto's disease are probably not at risk. But if you're sixty or older and have ever been diagnosed with Graves' or Hashimoto's disease, ask your doctor to specifically measure vitamin B_{12} levels in your blood. If the levels are low or borderline, request an additional test, known as the Schilling test, which can detect if you're having difficulty absorbing vitamin B_{12} from food. If you do have pernicious anemia, it is easily corrected with an intramuscular injection of vitamin B_{12}. Usually the treatment is once monthly, but, depending on the severity, it will vary.

Arthritis Some people with Graves' or Hashimoto's disease experience tendon and joint inflammation. Painful tendinitis and bursitis of the shoulder, for example, was reported in about 7 percent of Graves' and Hashimoto's patients, compared to only 1.7 percent of the general population.

On the other hand, rheumatoid arthritis, a more serious disease, appears to be only slightly more common among thyroid patients than the general population. Nevertheless, it can cause inflammation of many joints in the body including knuckles, wrists, and elbows. Stiffness tends to be more severe in the morning. If you are either hyper- or hypothyroid and have noticed this kind of pain or stiffness, ask your doctor to recommend appropriate medication for arthritic symptoms. Sometimes, pain and stiffness will improve when the thyroid condition is corrected.

Diabetes There is an increased incidence of Type 1 diabetes (a.k.a. juvenile diabetes or insulin-dependent diabetes) in families where Graves' or Hashimoto's disease has been diagnosed.

If you do happen to have both conditions, an overactive thyroid will often make the diabetes worse and more difficult to control with insulin. Once your thyroid condition is treated, though, you will regain control over the diabetes.

Addison's disease This is caused by your adrenal glands failing to make cortisone and steroid hormones—the adrenal "products" your body needs to function properly. This is rare among thyroid patients, *but* it tends to occur frequently in people with pernicious anemia, discussed above, which is commonly found in thyroid patients.

Inflammatory Bowel Disease (IBD) This is an umbrella term that comprises Crohn's disease as well as colitis. IBD is a miserable condition where the lower intestine becomes inflamed, causing abdominal cramping, pain, fever, and mucusy, bloody diarrhea. IBD occurs more often in thyroid disease patients and can generally be controlled through diet and medications. If you have IBD, it's best to ask to be referred to a gastroenterologist (a.k.a. G.I. specialist), who is the specialist to manage it. See my book, *The Gastrointestinal Sourcebook,* for details about IBD. This is not to be confused with irritable bowel syndrome (IBS), a stress-related disorder that often masks hyperthyroid symptoms. IBS is discussed on page 179.

Lupus This is a frightening condition that imitates many other diseases. For years, lupus patients went undiagnosed, similar to many thyroid patients. This is an autoimmune condition that affects many body tissues causing arthritic symptoms, skin rashes, and kidney, lung, and heart problems. Lupus patients often test positive for antithyroid antibodies. What's interesting about lupus is that it is rare among thyroid sufferers even though lupus sufferers often have thyroid problems. If you know someone with lupus, a thyroid function test is a good idea, which would at least relieve some of the symptoms.

Myasthenia gravis When I was doing a radio talk show one day about thyroid disease, a caller asked if I knew anything about this condition. I thought perhaps she was mispronouncing "Graves' disease" and feebly confessed complete ignorance. So I looked it up and guess what? It is a rare autoimmune disorder of the muscles that affects only about 30 people per 1 million, but it's *ten times* more common in Graves' disease patients. Symptoms include muscle weakness, double vision, and difficulty swallowing—symptoms that can be present in both Graves' and thyroid eye disease. What a nightmare if you should have both of them! So please ask to be tested for myasthenia gravis when you have these symptoms. They may *not* be caused solely by Graves' disease.

Other Stress-Related Disorders

Women suffering from thyroid disease are not immune to other stress-related disorders that can aggravate, or mask, thyroid symptoms. Two of the most common problems involve the urinary tract and the bowels.

Irritable Bowels?

A most confusing label has come into vogue that defines the bowel habits of between twenty-five to fifty-five million North Americans—two-thirds of which are women. The label is *irritable bowel syndrome* (IBS), which refers to unusual bowel "patterns" that alternate between diarrhea and constipation, and everything in between. IBS is also referred to as irritable or spastic colon; spastic, mucus, nervous, laxative, cathartic, or functional colitis; spastic bowel; nervous indigestion; functional dyspepsia; pylorospasm; and functional bowel disease. The problem with using the term *irritable* is that irritation is *not* what is transpiring. It also sounds too much like "inflammatory," which is not happening, either. Worse, many family doctors will say "IBS" instead of "We don't know what is going on—but have you tried fiber?"

The term *irritable bowel syndrome* came into use to describe a bowel that is overly sensitive to normal activity. In other words, when the nerve endings that line the bowel are too sensitive, the nerves controlling the gastrointestinal tract can become overactive, making the bowel overly responsive or "irritable" to normal things, such as the passing of gas or fluid. In other words, the bowel may want to pass a stool before it is ready. The bowel, in a sense, becomes too "touchy" for comfort. However, since we tend to think of irritable, when used clinically, as something that is red, irritated, or inflamed, this label is more confusing than defining. IBS has nothing to do with irritation, inflammation, or any organic disease process. It has to do with nerves.

The term *IBS* also implies that a diagnosis of your symptoms has been made and that there is a definite cause—and cure—for your condition. This is not true. IBS is a diagnosis made in the absence of any other diagnosis. There is no test to confirm IBS, only tests to rule out other causes for your symptoms. The term *functional bowel disorder* is beginning to catch on instead of IBS because "functional" means that there is no disease. Yet no matter what you call it, roughly half of all digestive disorders are attributed to IBS. After the common cold, IBS is the chief cause of absenteeism in the workplace. Many doctors compare IBS to asthma in that there are number of causes with the same outcome. Asthma may be related to allergies or a hundred other things. Similarly, IBS has many different causes that are difficult to pin down. Stress and dietary factors are the chief causes, however.

IBS symptoms IBS symptoms are characterized by frequent, violent episodes of diarrhea that will almost always strike around a stressful situation. (People often experience IBS symptoms before job interviews or plane trips.) Over 60 percent of IBS sufferers report that their symptoms first coincided with stressful events, while 40 to 60 percent of those with IBS also suffer from anxiety disorders or depression compared to 20 percent of people with other gastrointestinal disorders. Stressful events that can also trigger IBS include death of a loved one, separation/divorce, unresolved conflict or grief, moving to a new city or job, and having a history of childhood physical or sexual abuse.

Many people will find that their symptoms persist well beyond a stressful life event and that the episodes will invade their normal routine. There need not be one, single stressful event that precipitates IBS; it could first present itself after you've been in a stressful job over a long period of time or subjected to the normal stresses of "life in North America" for a period of time. Episodes of diarrhea are often accompanied by crampy, abdominal pains or gas, which are relieved by a bowel movement. The pain may shift around in the abdomen as well. After the diarrhea episodes subside, you may then be plagued by long bouts of constipation or the feeling that you're not emptying your bowels completely when you do go. Again, IBS refers to an irregular bowel *pattern* rather than one particular episode. The pattern is that there is no *normal* pattern of bowel movements; it is often one extreme or the other.

Your stools may also contain mucus, which can make the stool long and rope-like or worm-like. The mucus is normally secreted by the colon to help the stool along in a normal movement. In IBS, your colon secretes too much mucus.

Blood mixed with your stools means "This is not IBS, but something else, however." Some people can also suffer from solely diarrhea or solely gas, and constipation. Other symptoms include bloating, nausea, and loss of appetite. Fever, weight loss, or severe pain is not a sign of IBS but of something else.

Many people find it confusing that IBS can cause both constipation and diarrhea, which seem to be opposite ends of the spectrum. But what happens is that, instead of the slow muscular contractions that normally move the bowels, spasms occur, which can either result in an "explosion" or a "blockage." It can be compared to a sudden gust of wind: it can blow the door wide open (diarrhea) or blow it shut (constipation). It all depends on the direction of the wind at the time.

It's important to note the timing of your diarrhea; in IBS, your sleep should not be disturbed by it. The episodes will always occur either after a meal or in the early evening.

What distinguishes IBS from infectious diarrhea or inflammatory bowel diseases are:

- finding relief through defecation
- noticing looser stools when the bowel movement is precipitated by pain
- noticing more frequent bowel movements when you experience pain
- noticing abdominal bloating or distention
- noticing mucus in the stools
- feeling that you have not completely emptied your bowels

What to rule out The symptoms of IBS are obviously a little vague in that they can be signs of many other problems. Therefore, before you accept a diagnosis of IBS, make sure that your doctor has taken down your thorough medical history in order to further investigate:

- dietary culprits, food allergies, lactose intolerance, or just plain "poor diet"—high fats/starch; low fiber
- intestinal bacterial, viral, or parasitic infections (Where have you been traveling? What are your sexual habits?)
- overgrowth of *C. difficile,* a common cause of infectious diarrhea
- yeast in the gastrointestinal tract (called candidiasis), which is notorious for causing IBS symptoms (eating yogurt every day should clear this up)
- medications
- motility problems
- enzyme deficiencies (the pancreas may not be secreting enough enzymes to break down your food)
- serious disease such as inflammatory bowel or signs of cancer

Stress and IBS It's possible to have a pristine diet, to rule out all forms of organic disease, yet still suffer from IBS while under stress. In the same way that you can sweat, blush, or cry under emotional stress, your gastrointestinal tract may also react to stress by "weeping"—producing excessive water and mucus or overreacting to normal stimuli such as eating. What often happens, however, is that there is a delayed "gut reaction" to stress, meaning that you may not experience your IBS symptoms until your stress has passed. Apparently, your brain under stress becomes more active as a "defense mechanism." (For example, when we are running away from a predator, we have to think quickly and act quickly, so our heart rate increases, we perspire more, and so on). During this "defensive mode" the entire nervous system can become exaggerated (that's what causes "butterflies in the stomach"). The nerves controlling the gastrointestinal tract therefore become highly sensitive—which can cause IBS symptoms. Studies show, for example, that IBS symptoms are more common on weekday mornings than afternoons or weekends, while IBS symptoms do not appear at night while you are sleeping.

Women and IBS Why is IBS more common in women? For one thing, women menstruate and experience normal mood fluctuations related to their natural menstrual cycles. Mood changes are common premenstrual symptoms that may create more emotional stress, and, hence, IBS symptoms. Uterine contractions during menstruation constitutes another factor. When the uterus contracts, it often stimulates a bowel movement. The first day of a woman's period is often when she has several loose bowel movements. Meanwhile, a common symptom of labor is diarrhea and vomiting. This occurs because of the intensity of the uterine contractions that create "ripples" throughout the gastrointestinal tract.

Women who experience painful periods or endometriosis may also experience more intense IBS symptoms. In endometriosis, parts of the uterine lining grow outside of the uterus into the abdominal cavity, often triggering painful bowel movements, diarrhea, or constipation during or just prior to menstruation.

Finally, women are far more prone to eating disorders and laxative abuse as well as domestic abuse (resulting in continuous emotional upset and stress), all of which wreak havoc on the gastrointestinal tract.

Bladder Problems

Another stress-related condition women suffer from is interstitial cystitis (IC), which is the inflammation of the interstitium, the space between the bladder lining and bladder muscle. This can cause chronic pelvic pain, urinary frequency, and a shrunken, ulcerated bladder. The bladder itself is lined with a protective layer that is secreted, like mucus, by the cells that line the bladder. This layer protects the inside of the bladder from acids and toxins in the urine and prevents bacteria from sticking to the bladder wall. If this layer is damaged, as is the case with IC, infection can result.

IC symptoms include frequent urination (as many as sixty times per day). In addition, you may feel a bruising kind of pain around your clitoral area and find that acidic foods, chocolate, red wine, old cheese, nuts, yogurt, avocados, and bananas—and, sometimes, antibiotics—can make the pain worse. IC starts out as a normal urinary tract infection (known as bacterial cystitis). But, after a few bouts of cystitis, your urine cultures will all be negative.

There are several theories as to the causes of IC, including increased progesterone. In fact, postmenopausal women on progesterone may notice cystitis symptoms more than premenopausal women. If you have IC, you will need to see a urologist. There are numerous treatments that include anti-inflammatory drugs and bladder relaxants.

What Is Stress?

Since autoimmune disorders such as Graves' disease and Hashimoto's disease are believed to be triggered by stress, what can you do to manage your stress? Well, the first order of business is understanding what exactly stress is.

Generally, *stress* is defined as a negative emotional experience associated with biological changes that allow you to adapt to it. In response to stress, your adrenal glands pump out "stress hormones" that speed up your body: your heart rate increases and your blood sugar levels increase so that glucose can be diverted to your muscles in case you have to "run." This is known as the "fight or flight" response.

The problem with stress hormones in the twenty-first century is that the fight or flight response is not usually necessary since most of our stress is emotional. Occasionally, we may want to flee from a bank robbery or mugger, but most of us just want to flee from the stresses of daily life. In other words, our stress hormones actually put a physical strain on our bodies and can lower our resistance to disease. Initially, stress hormones stimulate our immune systems. But after the stressful event has passed, it can suppress the immune system and create a similar situation that results during pregnancy (see chapter 4).

Stress can affect every part of our body—from head to toe. We can suffer from stress-related:

- Headaches
- Gastrointestinal problems (read on)
- Bladder problems (read on)
- Cardiovascular problems
- Back pain
- High blood pressure
- High cholesterol

Good Stress

Good things can come from stress, too, even though it may feel "stressful" or bad in the short term. Stress challenges us to stretch ourselves beyond our capabilities, which is what makes us meet deadlines, push the "outside of the envelope," and invent creative solutions to our problems. Examples of good stress include challenging projects; positive life-changing events (moving, changing jobs, or ending unhealthy relationships); confronting fears, illness, or people who make us feel bad (this is bad in the short-term, good in the long-term situation). Essentially, whenever a stressful event triggers emotional, intellectual, or spiritual growth, it is "good stress." It is often not the event as much as it is your *response* to the event that determines whether it is "good" or "bad" stress. The death of a loved one can sometimes lead to personal growth because we may learn something about ourselves we did not see before—a new inner resilience, for example. So even the death of a loved one can constitute "good stress" even though we grieve and are sad in the short term.

Bad Stress

Bad stress can result from boredom and stagnation. When no growth occurs from the stressful event, it is "bad stress." When negative events do not seem to yield anything positive in the long term, but instead more of the same, the stress can lead to chronic and debilitating health problems. This is not to say that we can't get sick from "good stress," either. Rather, it is to say that when there are no positive elements to be gleaned from the stress, it will have a much more negative impact on our health. Some examples of bad stress include stagnant jobs or relationships, disability from terrible accidents or diseases, or long-term unemployment. These kind of situations can lead to depression, low self-esteem, and a host of physical illnesses.

Women's Stress

A variety of unique stresses exist for women. They include:

- *Violence.* At least half of all women have experienced domestic violence.
- *Poverty.* Single women and women of color are far more likely to live in poverty than white men. After a divorce, a man's income will increase by roughly 20 percent, yet a woman's income will decrease by at least 50 percent.
- *Workplace stress and/or harassment.* This is frequently underreported and creates significant stress for women.
- *Beauty standards.* Oppressive or even impossible standards of beauty is another factor that makes life difficult for women.
- *Hormonal factors.* Hormonal changes related to the menstrual cycle, pregnancy, postpartum changes, and menopause add stress to women's lives.

Managing Stress

What we perceive as stressful often has great bearing on how well we manage it. Women that are already overloaded will feel added stress as well. In general, we feel stress when we experience:

- Negative events
- Uncontrollable or unpredictable events
- Ambiguous events (versus clear-cut situations)

Thyroid disease meets all three criteria. And how stressed you become has much to do with your personality as well. For example, if you have a negative outlook on life, you will probably feel more stress than someone with a positive outlook. Some women like to find meaning in uncontrollable events in order to give them a sense of control. Others like the challenge of difficult situations.

Our strategies for coping also vary. Some women like to avoid stress in order to minimize a problem. This has short-term benefits, but in the long term the stress does not disappear. Women who confront stress in the short term will feel more anxious at first but then (probably) feel relief in the long term once the stress is dealt with. People who suffer less stress-related health problems use humor, spiritual support, and social support to deal with stress.

Stress Reduction

Because so many of the health problems discussed in this chapter are manifestations of stress, what can you do to lower your stress—realistically? Being told to simply "take things easy" and "relax" is not a solution, because, indeed, if we weren't so stressed, we would relax!

Stress reduction depends entirely on the source of stress. The only way to manage stress that is beyond your control is to shift your response. And for many women, this takes time and may require some work with a qualified counselor.

If you are the source of your own stress because you're too hard on yourself or are a perfectionist, you need to work on lowering your self-expectations and forgiving yourself for not being perfect. Again, working with a therapist or counselor may help. In the meantime, here are suggestions for reducing some sources of daily stress:

1. Isolate the exact source of stress and see if there's a solution. (Taking the time to think about what, in fact, the real problem is can work wonders.)

2. See the humor in difficult situations, and try to look at lessons learned instead of beating yourself up.
3. When times get tough, surround yourself with supportive people: close friends, family members, etc.
4. Do not take things so personally. When people do not respond to you the way you would like, consider other factors. For instance, maybe the other person has problems unrelated to you that are affecting his or her behavior.
5. Focus on something pleasant in the future, such as a vacation, and allow yourself time to daydream, plan, and so on.
6. Just say "No." If you cannot take on that "small favor" or extra task, just politely say "I would love to, but it is just not possible now."
7. Take time out for yourself. Spend some time alone and block everyone out once a week or so. This is a great time to just go for a long walk and get in a little exercise.
8. Lists. Some people find that making lists really helps; others find that it is just another "chore" in and of itself. If you have never been a listmaker, try it. It might help you to get a bit more focused and organized for tackling the tasks at hand.
9. Investigate alternative healing systems, such as massage, and Chinese exercises, such as qi gong (pronounced "chi kong") or tai chi.
10. Eat properly.

A Little Hedonism Goes a Long Way

I know this will sound glib and trite and torn from the pages of the latest fluff magazine, but many women report that small pleasures can help them unwind. If you have children, try to schedule some of the following at least once every couple of weeks. You probably know about them already, but here is a reminder nonetheless:

1. *Aromatherapy.* Who cares if it doesn't have the medicinal benefits that it claims! It smells nice and makes you feel pampered and special. Splurge on a decanter, buy some tea

lights, take a bath, turn the lights off, and soak up the atmosphere for twenty minutes.

2. *Take a bath anyway.* Bubble baths are important. (If you have sensitive skin, ask a dermatologist or family doctor to recommend something that will soothe your skin.) Many women make this a nightly ritual. If you really want to be decadent, take a glass of wine or favorite food into the tub with you!

3. *Modern meditation.* Okay—so not everyone can get into meditating properly, complete with chants and incense. Here's a compromise: Put on your favorite music, turn out the lights, and light a candle. It's amazing what this can do for your mental health.

4. *Go for a walk around the block without thinking about it as exercise.* Take a leisurely "stroll," not a brisk walk that gets your heart rate up. This is a great way to just let your mind wander and recharge your batteries.

5. *Have a chick-flick night!* Whether it's seeing *Gone With The Wind* for the fiftieth time or salivating over your favorite male or female lead, get decadent. Make popcorn, fondue, or whatever turns you on. The rule is not to feel guilty about spending time slumbering in front of the VCR.

Few things can be more stressful than sweating out the investigation of a "lump." The next chapter discusses benign lumps on the thyroid gland and thyroid cancer, as well as thyroid surgery and treatment with radioactive iodine.

CHAPTER 9

Thyroid Lumps and Thyroid Cancer

Approximately 10 percent of the population will develop nodules on the thyroid gland, yet only 5 percent of these nodules will ever turn out to be thyroid cancer. Even so, there are about 14,000 new cases of thyroid cancer each year in the U.S., and about 1,000 deaths. Women outnumber men in developing thyroid cancer by 3 to 1. Put another way, women account for 77 percent of all new cases of thyroid cancer, and 61 percent of all deaths.

What makes thyroid cancer uniquely a "woman's issue" is that we now know that it is caused largely by radiation exposure and radioactive fallout. From the 1940s through the 1960s, many women were exposed to radiation as children because they may have received treatment to their head and neck areas for acne. Women were treated more often than men for cosmetic reasons. Because women have more fat on their bodies than men, they are also more vulnerable to radiation exposure than men; thus they are more likely to develop cancer. Although radiation exposure is also linked to breast cancer, no one disputes the fact that thyroid cancer is an environmental cancer, while there are still plenty of experts who deny the link of radiation to breast cancer.

Right now, the National Cancer Institute recommends that anyone who received radiation treatments to the head or neck in childhood be examined by a doctor every one to two years.

Investigating a Thyroid Lump

A lump is called a "nodule," which literally means "knot" and refers to a lump that can vary from the size of a pea to the size of a golf ball. Single thyroid nodules are usually one of three things: a growth that contains fluid (called a cyst), a growth that contains lazy, abnormal cells (called a benign tumor or adenoma), or a growth that contains active abnormal cells (called an adenocarcinoma).

Cysts containing fluid are always benign. A needle biopsy immediately and easily determines whether or not the lump has fluid. A needle biopsy means that the doctor will stick a long needle into the lump and suck out whatever fluid is inside. The fluid is then biopsied, or investigated. This procedure is about as uncomfortable as getting a flu shot or giving blood. However, when the lump is not a cyst, it can prove the difference between lazy and active abnormal cells which makes a lump benign or malignant.

An adenoma involves glandular cells, which usually clump together in a harmless, benign lump. Because the thyroid is a gland, any benign tumor that develops on it is called an adenoma. When abnormal cells grow on the thyroid gland they vary in activity. Sometimes the cells are like "bumps on a log"; they are lazy, inactive, and just "there" without a purpose. It is as though the cells develop and then lack the drive or capability to do anything else. They don't reproduce, don't imitate other thyroid cells, and don't interfere with normal thyroid function. They simply exist. These cells live in a clump and appear as a nodule on or around your thyroid. When they're investigated, they're considered benign (i.e., harmless), which means that the lump is noncancerous. This is an adenoma.

Adenocarcinoma   The word *carcinoma* refers to a malignant (i.e., cancerous) growth that involves the epithelial cells, or cells which line the surface of our insides. But when a tumor in a glandular area is malignant, and stems from these epithelial cells, it's referred to as an adenocarcinoma.

When abnormal cells develop, they are often far more active and purposeful. Sometimes they spend all of their time reproducing. Or they may spend only half their time reproducing and the other half assisting or mimicking normal thyroid cells. They also live in clumps and appear as a nodule on or around your thyroid gland. When these cells are investigated, they are discovered to be malignant, which means that the lump is cancerous. This is an adenocarcinoma. It is these active, abnormal cells that pose a threat to the rest of your body. Given the opportunity, they will mass produce themselves and invade, or "metastasize," to other parts of the body. (The word *metastasis* means invasion.) That's why it's very important to diagnose this condition as early as possible. Generally, the harder the lump is, the more likely it is to be malignant. A softer, fleshier lump tends to be benign.

Solitary toxic adenoma There is another kind of benign growth known as a solitary toxic adenoma. Here, either a clump of cells or a singular growth develops and takes over all thyroid gland function. The adenoma is toxic in this case because it causes hyperthyroidism. The adenoma basically "hijacks" the main gland and assumes full production of thyroid hormone. The pituitary gland, which regulates thyroid stimulating hormone, gets confused by the situation and turns off. What happens then is that there is no monitoring system in place, and the adenoma makes too much thyroid hormone. This is common in middle-aged or elderly patients. A solitary toxic adenoma is a type of thyroid disorder and is not malignant. It is easily treated via thyroid replacement hormone which deactivates the growth.

Diagnosing Lumps

A diagnostic procedure known as fine needle aspiration (FNA) has changed the way thyroid lumps are diagnosed. If you walked into your doctor's office with a lump on your neck five years ago, you may have had the entire lump removed through a procedure known as excisional biopsy—a nasty little procedure that was used to diagnose my own thyroid cancer. You also may have been sent for an ultrasound to determine if your lump was fluid-filled or solid. These procedures are rarely necessary today.

FNA, a twenty-minute procedure, is basically considered the gold standard now for evaluating a thyroid nodule. It can be performed in a doctor's office and is as simple as drawing a blood sample. The skin around your lump is cleansed with antiseptic, and some doctors inject a local anesthetic into the site before doing FNA. Many patients don't want or need this, however. The needle (which is smaller than the standard needles used to sample blood) needs to be inserted three to six times to obtain a good sample, and sucks out cells and/or fluid (the latter if it's a cyst), which is then sent off to a pathologist (a specialist who examines cells), who is then able to determine if the lump is benign or malignant (see Figure 9.1). FNA is accurate four out of five times. If your lump is a cyst, this procedure can also drain and collapse it, taking care of the problem entirely. The benefits of FNA outweigh other diagnostic procedures because it is cheap, easy, fast, accurate, and places far less stress on you, the patient.

Studies show that since the introduction of FNA, thyroid surgery has dropped by 50 percent. This means that many people can be spared "look-see surgery" (which used to be performed frequently when cancer was suspected). The end result is that while the number of thyroid cancers have not substantially increased (in North America anyway), only half as many people today require thyroid cancer surgery.

If there's any question about the diagnosis, or your doctor wants to get a *structural* picture of what's going on, you might be referred for a thyroid scan (discussed under "Hot Versus Cold Nodules" on page 196).

Ultrasound may be used to check structure, too, but this basically has been abandoned in thyroid nodule testing because of FNA. At one time ultrasound was useful because it told doctors whether the lump was hollow (a sign of a cyst) or solid. But today, ordering an ultrasound to evaluate thyroid nodules wouldn't give much information. You may want to request FNA if it's not offered or at least ask *why* it's not being offered (there may be a good reason). For example, many doctors aren't trained in the FNA procedure, while smaller communities may not have a pathologist trained to read the samples obtained through FNA.

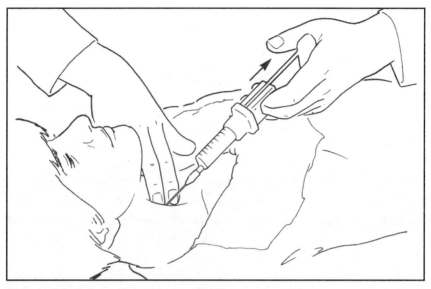

Figure 9.1 Fine needle aspiration (FNA).
Reprinted from *Nichts Gutes im Schilde Krankheiten der Schiddruse.* Copyright 1994, Georg Thieme Publishing.

Other types of needle biopsies Something known as a core needle biopsy (a.k.a. cutting needle biopsy) is the "parent" of FNA. A core needle biopsy will be done if FNA is not available. This procedure is exactly the same except that a larger needle is used and a larger amount of thyroid tissue is obtained, which necessitates the use of a local anesthetic. Core needle biopsies are also done in a hospital on an outpatient basis and may cause a little more bleeding and bruising from the puncture site.

Preparing for needle biopsies: Before and after Any time you have either FNA or core needle biopsy, it's a good idea to avoid medications that prolong blood clotting, such as aspirin, ibuprofen, etc. If you're on prescription medication, let your doctor know this prior to the procedure. However, being on these medications doesn't mean you can't have this done—it just reduces the risk of bleeding. Once the procedure is done the puncture site will be bandaged and you can go home. You may have some neck tenderness or mild swelling afterward, but you'll be fine within twenty-four hours. If you develop a fever or begin bleeding, get yourself to a doctor or emergency room quickly; this may be a sign of infection at the puncture site.

Lobectomy and Thyroidectomy

When the lump is located on or within the thyroid gland itself, and the surgeon even suspects the possibility of a malignancy, more serious surgery that requires you to be under a general anesthetic will be performed. Depending on where the lump is positioned, and its size, you may need only part of the gland removed. This is called a lobectomy (the thyroid gland is divided into two lobes), or partial thyroidectomy. Often, a good portion of the thyroid gland is removed under these circumstances, or a total thyroidectomy (removal of the thyroid gland) is performed. There is some controversy as to whether a lobectomy should be performed at all when a lump is suspicious. Read on for details.

Hot Versus Cold Nodules

Often, instead of a blood test prior to a biopsy, a thyroid scan is done. This is an imaging test that photographs the structure of your thyroid gland. It also involves a tracer of radioactive iodine. A twenty-four-hour test, its purpose in this case is to check for suspicious nodules. Normally your thyroid gland absorbs iodine to make thyroid hormone. But when your thyroid gland is abnormal, radioactive iodine is absorbed (see chapter 10 for more details). So, in essence, a radioactive iodine scan measures how abnormal your thyroid structure is.

For day 1 of the test, you are given a tiny amount of radioactive iodine and then sent home. On day 2 (twelve hours later) you return to the hospital where an imager takes photographs, or images, of your thyroid gland, which has now had time to absorb the radioactive iodine. Your doctor can tell how suspicious the lumps are by how much iodine they have absorbed.

A newer tracer, called technetium, can also be used. Widely used in many hospitals, you are given a tiny amount of technetium and wait just two hours for your scan. This tracer is obviously far more convenient.

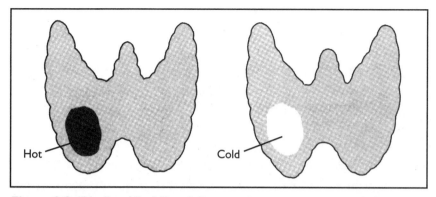

Figure 9.2 "Hot" and "cold" nodules.
Reprinted from *Nichts Gutes im Schilde Krankheiten der Schiddruse*. Copyright 1994, Georg Thieme Publishing.

A "hot" nodule is a lump on the thyroid gland consisting of functioning thyroid cells. Therefore, these lumps absorb the radioactive iodine eagerly because the cells inside are intelligent enough to recognize iodine. Chances are, if the nodule is functioning, or "hot," it is not cancerous. In these cases, the lump that is found is either one of the nodules comprising a multinodular goiter (described below) or is a solitary toxic adenoma (described above).

A "cold" nodule, on the other hand, consists of more primitive cells that lack the intelligence to recognize and hence absorb iodine. (See Figure 9.2.) A cold nodule is therefore more suspicious—and more likely to be cancerous. However, only 10 percent of all cold nodules found turn out to be malignant. A cold nodule means simply that the cells making up the nodule are abnormal and primitive. But it is the activity of these primitive cells that has yet to be determined—and that can only be done through a biopsy. If your scan shows the presence of hot nodules only, your doctor will probably not bother to do a biopsy because cancerous cells are never hot. If your scan shows the presence of either a cold nodule, or a mixture of hot and cold nodules (usually the case with a multinodular goiter), a biopsy is always done to investigate whether the cold nodules are malignant or benign. A cold nodule merely means that it is a suspicious nodule, not necessarily cancerous. Only a biopsy can determine with certainty whether a cold nodule is cancerous.

Benign Thyroid Nodules

Your medical history, age, and sex often determine the likelihood of benign or malignant tumors. Older people usually develop benign nodules as their bodies age; natural wear and tear has much to do with this. Similarly, if you are an adult woman, it's far more likely that your nodule is benign; adult women, as a rule, retain more water and have more fat on their bodies than men. This is because women need the extra fat to menstruate and bear children. As a result, benign lumps can often occur, particularly around the breasts. Furthermore, older women are more likely to have benign tumors on their thyroids than younger women. In addition, if you come from a family with a history of Hashimoto's disease, or multinodular goiters, your lump is also likely to be benign.

Another sign of a benign nodule is whether you are suffering from hypothyroidism or hyperthyroidism, or have in fact developed a goiter in addition to the nodule. If you present symptoms of either condition (or both—as is sometimes the case with Hashimoto's disease), your nodule is probably benign and is most likely a by-product of a defined thyroid disorder of some kind. For example, hyperthyroidism is caused by toxic adenomas or multinodular goiters. Or thyroiditis can sometimes cause lumps on the thyroid gland.

A lump is usually benign if you discover more than one, or if the rest of the thyroid gland itself is enlarged or irregular in some way. Benign lumps also tend to be fleshier, softer, and can sometimes shrink slightly in size from one examination to the next. In fact, when a doctor first examines a lump, he or she will usually do nothing and ask you to come back in a couple of weeks. That way, the doctor can see if the lump has changed in size at all (which is often the case). If it shrinks slightly, it's almost always benign; if it grows, it's more suspicious.

Multinodular Goiter

The good news is that when you have more than one lump on your thyroid gland, the lumps are usually benign and are there for a different reason. The term *multinodular* means "many nodules," as is the case with a multinodular goiter. What happens here is that lumps form on your thyroid gland, mimicking the gland in every conceivable way.

These nodules watch the thyroid gland in action and in time learn to make T3 and T4—thyroid hormone—as well. The nodules are completely unaware of the pituitary gland, which by contrast is aware of the intruding nodules. As a warning to the thyroid gland, the pituitary gland appropriately shuts off TSH secretion, which alerts the thyroid gland to slow down production. And it does. But T3 and T4 are still produced in uncontrolled quantities from the copycat nodules. The result is an enlarged thyroid gland and hyperthyroidism, known as a toxic multinodular goiter. At first, the goiter and the hyperthyroidism may suggest Graves' disease, but a doctor can usually feel that the goiter in this case is lumpy. Multinodular goiters tend to occur in postmenopausal women, while Graves' disease flourishes in premenopausal women. In addition, thyroid eye disease does not occur with a toxic multinodular goiter. So the absence of certain symptoms, coupled with your age, is often a strong indicator of the cause of your goiter.

If a multinodular goiter is diagnosed, usually a thyroid biopsy is done to rule out the possibility of a malignant nodule. You may be given thyroid replacement hormone if the nodules are not overactive which, in theory, should shrink the gland and hence the nodules. But often the multinodular goiter and nodules will not shrink. If the goiter is really out of control (for example, it may continue to enlarge to the point where your windpipe is compressed) and you don't respond to thyroid replacement hormone, your thyroid may be surgically removed, which would solve the problem. Then you would be put on thyroid replacement hormone permanently. Many studies are now showing that radioactive iodine therapy is a more effective way of shrinking *nontoxic* multinodular goiters (multinodular goiters that do *not* cause hyperthyroidism). In these cases, thyroid hormone replacement doesn't seem to work.

Thyroid Cancer

While most malignant thyroid lumps are hard and painless, some signs exist which indicate that a lump may be malignant. For example, if your lump continues to enlarge while you're on thyroid hormone, this is a clue that it's cancerous; thyroid hormone usually shrinks benign lumps. If you notice pain in your neck tissues, jawbone, or ear, or have difficulty swallowing food or liquids, wheeze, or have hoarseness, this may indicate that the cancer is spreading beyond the thyroid gland.

Since the 1940s, thyroid cancer has been completely treatable 95 percent of the time. First, thyroid cancer is a particularly lazy kind of cancer that grows slowly and takes a very long time to spread. In fact, you could conceivably walk around with undiagnosed thyroid cancer for a decade and still respond well to treatment. Second, radioactive iodine (discovered in the 1940s) will often eradicate thyroid cancer. In a way, radioactive iodine is frequently a miracle treatment for thyroid cancer.

About 10 percent of all thyroid patients are diagnosed with thyroid cancer in which abnormal, primitive cells have developed on the thyroid gland and are actively reproducing. Unless these cells are removed or killed off somehow, they will eventually spread and invade (or metastasize) other parts of your body. When these invasions or metastases occur, they interfere with normal bodily functions. In the worst-case scenario, thyroid cancer could spread to the bones or lungs. (It might take twenty years, but it's possible.) If that were to happen, then, yes—thyroid cancer could be fatal. But the truth is, more women die today during childbirth than from thyroid cancer. If you have the misfortune of developing cancer, the thyroid gland might just be the best place to get it; it is the most *curable* form of cancer.

Thyroid cancer is usually caught in a primary or secondary stage. In the primary stage, a malignant nodule or lump is found on the thyroid gland. In the secondary stage, a malignant nodule is found in a lymph node nearby, which is traced to the thyroid gland. Therefore, in a secondary stage, the thyroid cancer has already spread beyond the thyroid gland. In my own case, my thyroid cancer was discovered in a secondary stage, which is generally about as severe as it gets for the average thyroid cancer patient.

Radioactive Fallout and Thyroid Cancer

Radioactive iodine is emitted whenever fallout from nuclear accidents, testing, and, of course, atomic bomb tests occurs. Sadly, we are witnessing a tremendous increase in childhood thyroid cancer in certain "hot" areas, particularly areas in Russia, Balarus, and the Ukraine that were exposed to fallout from the 1986 Chernobyl nuclear reactor accident that released 40 million curies (a unit of measurement) of radioactive iodine into the atmosphere. That's a lot, considering Graves' disease patients (see chapter 8) receive 10 millicuries ($1/100$th of a curie) in treatment and thyroid cancer patients 100 millicuries.

The Chernobyl nuclear accident exposed millions of people with healthy thyroid glands to excessive levels of radioactive iodine. People living within a 30 km zone of the accident inhaled the radioactive iodine, while people living outside the 30 km zone were exposed to the radioactive iodine. For reasons not quite understood, potassium iodide (discussed on page 212) was not distributed to any of these people. Now, there appears to be a *twentyfold* increase in the incidence of thyroid cancer in children, in Belarus, Russia, and the Ukraine. For example, in one study conducted in the Ukraine between 1981 and 1985, the number of new cases of thyroid cancer in children up to age fourteen totaled twenty-five. But between 1986 and 1994, the number of new cases of thyroid cancer totaled 210, with peak periods occurring from 1992 to 1993.

Reports of high rates of thyroid cancer have also been documented from Hanford, Washington, where residents were exposed to fallout from the Hanford nuclear facility which produced plutonium for nuclear weapons from 1944 through 1957. If you live in that area, a new program offers estimates of radiation doses to Hanford "downwinders." You can receive an estimate of the amount of radioactive iodine 131 that your thyroid was exposed to during that period by calling 1-800-432-6242.

Anyone living downwind from the Nevada Test Site (residents in southwestern Utah, for example) between 1951 and 1962 are also vulnerable to thyroid cancer. A fourteen-year National Cancer Institute study published in 1997 examined the health risks from radioactive fallout released at the Nevada Test Site from 1951 to 1958. The conclusions reached stated that people living in the midwestern regions of North America may be more at risk for thyroid cancer, particularly if they were children at the time of testing.

Other areas affected by fallout include the Marshall Islands in the South Pacific—a result of atomic bomb testing at Bikini Atoll in

1954. There, thyroid cancers have occurred one hundred times more frequently than in the general population.

In the aftermath of the very long Cold War, more information is slowly becoming available about just how "hot" North America, Europe, and other parts of the world really are. The predictions are that incidences of thyroid cancer will continue to rise during our lifetime. We are witnessing similar trends in other cancers, too.

The North Dakota State Health Department reported in 1994 that the incidence of thyroid cancer in that state had doubled from 5 to 10 percent. The increase was attributed to radioactive iodine fallout. The Oak Ridge Health Agreement Steering Panel reported that young women born in 1952 who drank contaminated milk produced in test fallout areas were more likely to develop thyroid cancer in their lifetime than women born in the northeastern U.S.

The U.S. Energy Research Foundation concluded that there may be thousands of North Americans who ingested milk that was contaminated from this fallout and who are at greater risk for thyroid cancer.

Thyroid cancer may not be the only consequence of radioactive fallout. For example, the *Nashville Tennessean,* a daily newspaper, investigated "mysterious" illnesses afflicting people working at and living near nuclear weapons plants and research facilities from California to New York. Not only was there a high incidence of thyroid cancer but also a high incidence of autoimmune diseases, including autoimmune thyroid diseases. Workers around nuclear facilities in Tennessee, Ohio, Kentucky, Colorado, South Carolina, New Mexico, Idaho, New York, California, Texas, and Washington all reported the same trend. For more information, visit the newspaper's Web site at www.tennessean.com.

The Asia-California Phenomenon

Another group at risk for thyroid cancer are Asian women who have immigrated to California. Studies have only just begun, but researchers suspect that there exists a link between nutritional factors and iodine. The theory is that, somehow, when these women changed from an iodine-deficient diet as young women to an iodine-rich diet as an adult or older woman, the change in iodine content triggered thyroid cancer. These women are being tracked by an examination of their toenail clippings which, apparently constitute a good marker for trace elements.

X-ray Therapy

In the 1940s and 1950s, X-ray therapy was commonly used to treat infants with enlarged thymus glands (falsely believed to cause crib death) and children with enlarged adenoids and tonsils. X-ray therapy was also used to treat facial acne in teenagers, birthmarks, whooping cough, scalp ringworm, and sometimes as a means to try to stimulate hearing in the deaf. The practice of using X-ray began in the 1920s, peaked in the 1940s and 1950s, and slowly petered out in the 1960s. The treatment involved an X-ray machine (called external beam irradiation) or placing radioactive material like radium directly in or on the tissue to be treated. The immediate results were often promising. For example, acne improved, while acne scarring was reduced and some forms of deafness were improved. (Enlarged lymph tissue would sometimes block the inner ear and cause deafness; radiation was used to shrink the lymph tissue and thus improve hearing.)

The long-term consequences of X-ray treatment canceled out any short-term benefits, however. Unlike laser treatment, X-ray treatment couldn't be concentrated onto one small area without irradiating surrounding areas. Since the thyroid gland is located in the center of the neck, X-ray beamed at the face (acne), adenoids, tonsils, thymus gland, ears, or scalp were also targeting the thyroid gland. By the 1950s, doctors began to notice an increase in benign and malignant nodules on the thyroid glands of patients who had been treated previously with X-ray. Then, by the late 1950s and early 1960s, it was discovered that many victims of the atomic bombings in Hiroshima and Nagasaki were developing malignant tumors on their thyroid glands. When these reports became public, doctors concluded that radiation was the cause. X-ray treatments were subsequently banned.

It's estimated that millions of people throughout North America, Europe, and the U.K. received these treatments. (In the U.S., over two million people alone are estimated.) Generally, nodules have been discovered anywhere from ten to sixty years later in people who received X-ray therapy in the past. Usually, though, people are vulnerable between the ages of thirty to fifty. If you have received these treatments or suspect that you may have (often, children were too young and naive to realize they were receiving X-ray, or the treatment was given to infants), get your thyroid checked regularly—at least once a year, and tell your doctor why you want your thyroid examined. Or, if you can remember where you lived when you received X-ray treatment, you can contact the hospitals in that area and request your medical records. If your childhood doctor is still alive, find out where your old records are. Often when doctors retire, they turn over their entire practice to younger doctors, who often keep old records. (Usually, records are kept anywhere from twenty-five to fifty years.) To request old records, contact the Medical Records Department of the hospital or ask for the Medical Records Librarian on duty. You will want to ask what kind of treatment you received and how much radiation was used. Sometimes, hospitals will take the initiative and contact you by mail to inform you of such treatments. If you are contacted, see your doctor and arrange to have your thyroid checked regularly.

Types of Thyroid Cancer

Thyroid cancer is divided into two categories: differentiated and undifferentiated. These terms refer to the sophistication of the cancer cells. Differentiated cancer cells act and look like normal thyroid cells. In fact, they actually assist the other cells with routine functions such as making thyroxine. Because these cells spend time assisting the thyroid gland, they spend less time reproducing and therefore take a lot longer to metastasize to other parts of the body. Differentiated cancer such as this is the most common form of thyroid cancer. The cancer is more specifically referred to as a papillary cancer or follicular cancer.

Papillary and follicular refer to both the physical shape and personality of the cancer cells, as well as their behavior. In essence, if papillary is blonde and passive, follicular is brunette and aggressive. In other words, follicular is a more dangerous or active kind of cancer. However, it's very common for the cells to be a combination of papillary and follicular. This is called a papillary follicular mix. When this happens, the passive, more "reasonable" papillary cancer counteracts some of the aggressiveness of the follicular cancer. For this reason, this kind of cancer is extremely treatable and affords the patient an excellent survival rate. In fact, a papillary follicular mix is the most common type of thyroid cancer. For women under fifty and men under forty, the cure rate is just about 100 percent. In a worst-case scenario, this cancer has only a 17 percent chance of recurrence, and a history of only a 1.7 percent death rate. Papillary tumors account for about 60 percent of all thyroid cancers; only about 1 percent of all thyroid cancers will be follicular tumors.

When thyroid cancer is purely papillary, it's obviously far less aggressive than a type that is purely follicular. But the survival rate for both is still excellent; for women under fifty and men under forty, it's almost 100 percent. Papillary and follicular cancers tend to occur in younger people anyway (i.e., under age forty). Hurthle cell cancer, an even more aggressive form of follicular cancer, is the type of thyroid cancer that generally occurs in people over sixty. But because it is differentiated, this cancer is also very treatable.

Undifferentiated cancer is comprised of very primitive cells that spend all their time reproducing. This is a very rare but more severe form of thyroid cancer, called anaplastic cancer. Anaplastic cancer cells therefore spread faster because they contribute nothing to the thyroid gland; their existence is devoted solely to reproduction. This cancer is almost never found in patients under age forty and is usually discovered in elderly patients. The survival rate from anaplastic cancer is not good, and it is usually not treatable. Roughly 18 percent of all thyroid cancers are anaplastic. It generally occurs in women over age sixty.

There is also an inherited thyroid cancer called medullary cancer, which accounts for one out of ten cases of thyroid cancer. Here, a specific cell that secretes a hormone called calcitonin takes up residence in your thyroid gland. This cell is called a "C" cell and can actually be detected through a specific blood test that checks for calcitonin. If medullary thyroid cancer runs in your family, you would be alerted either by other family members or by a doctor familiar with your family history. Then, your blood would be checked for calcitonin about once a year. Medullary cancer is less severe than anaplastic but is more serious than differentiated cancers. It is still quite treatable, though. Recently, a blood test was developed by a University of Michigan doctor, which is considered a breakthrough in medullary thyroid cancer. Though it affects only about 1,000 people in the U.S. annually (i.e., a tiny segment of the population), this test can detect a *specific* gene that places you at risk for this kind of cancer. So if you tested positive for the medullary thyroid cancer gene, you would have what's called a "prophylactic thyroidectomy," meaning a preventive thyroidectomy. This removes the risk of *ever* developing medullary thyroid cancer, a type that can spread and develop into more serious cancer.

Finally, the presence of cancer cells on your thyroid gland can mean that cancer originating elsewhere has spread to your thyroid gland. In this case, the cancer would not be thyroid cancer at all but an invading cancer that comes from a different place in your body, like a kidney or breast. If this were the case, the origin of this metastatic, or spreading, cancer would have been detected long before it reached your thyroid gland.

Treating Thyroid Cancer

The usual treatment scenario involves a combination of surgery and radioactive iodine therapy. Sometimes, when the cancer is in a secondary stage, you will need radiation therapy (discussed on page 209.) However, only if you had a rare, undifferentiated, or anaplastic form of thyroid cancer would you require chemotherapy. Thyroid cancer generally has a very low recurrence rate. For most age groups, and with most forms of thyroid cancer, the cancer only recurs about 17 percent of the time.

Surgery Regardless of what stage your cancer is in, surgery is almost always used as a form of treatment. Even if your cancer was detected from a lump on the thyroid gland, which means the cancer has not

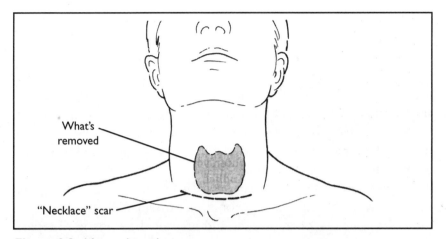

Figure 9.3 After a thyroidectomy.
Reprinted from *Nichts Gutes im Schilde Krankheiten der Schiddruse.* Copyright 1994, Georg Thieme Publishing.

spread beyond your thyroid gland and is therefore in a primary stage, a total or near total thyroidectomy is still performed. "Why take chances?" is the prevailing philosophy.

When thyroid cancer is detected from a lump in the neck, it means that your thyroid cancer is in a secondary stage. Here, the cancer has spread beyond your thyroid gland to the surrounding lymph nodes in your neck. In this case you will need to have your entire thyroid gland removed as well as the surrounding lymph nodes. This is called a total thyroidectomy (see Figure 9.3). The surgeon will also want to examine seemingly healthy lymph nodes further in the neck to ensure there is no cancer present. To do this, a few lymph nodes will be removed and, while you are still in surgery, quickly examined under a microscope to determine if any thyroid cells are present. If there are, it means that the cancer has spread a little further into the neck and the surgeon will remove all lymph tissue having thyroid cells. This is called a neck dissection.

Only in rarer forms of thyroid cancer is surgery not recommended. Surgery, however, is always the first stage of treatment for differentiated forms of thyroid cancer.

Total thyroidectomy versus a partial thyroidectomy (a.k.a. lobectomy) is an extremely controversial issue at present with thyroid surgeons and endocrinologists. Many surgeons take the "conservation" approach: they want to leave as much thyroid tissue intact as possible. While very noble, according to the best studies and top surgeons, this is generally the *wrong* approach when thyroid cancer has been detected—even if it's small and localized. Given that there is even a small chance that thyroid cancer can recur, or that a surgeon may not be able to detect every cancerous tidbit, radioactive iodine therapy is usually recommended to "finish the job." The only time lobectomy is acceptable is if you have a papillary cancer less than 1 cm in size or if a highly noninvasive follicular cancer is present. Clearly, it may be worth having a total thyroidectomy in this situation to absolutely minimize your risk of recurrence and prevent the scenario of repeat thyroid surgery (I know people who have been through it!).

Radioactive iodine therapy following a thyroidectomy is an important way to eradicate all thyroid tissue—and, hence, potentially cancerous tissue. It is also an important way to detect recurrence of thyroid cancer. But if there is half a thyroid gland still left inside you, radioactive iodine therapy will not be all that effective because it will probably wind up causing thyroiditis (this happens about 60 percent of the time). And a radioactive iodine scan is useless because it's designed to pick up thyroid remnants that can't be seen with the naked eye. The bottom line is that the more thyroid tissue that is left inside you, the more potential there is for it to become cancerous and, hence, necessitate a repeat of all diagnostic tests as well as surgery.

If you do have a lobectomy, you may not require any thyroid hormone after surgery. The remaining lobe usually enlarges slightly and works "double time" to produce enough hormone for your body.

Risks of surgery With an experienced surgeon who does at least one thyroidectomy a week, the risks of surgery are minimal. At any rate, about 1 percent of thyroidectomy patients will experience damage to nerves leading to the voice box, which is located very close to the thyroid. There may also be some damage to the parathyroid glands, which, as discussed in chapter 1, control calcium levels. Damage can cause numbness and tingling sensations around the lips, mouth, hands, and feet. Muscle cramps and twitching, and sometimes even seizures, can occur as well. If this happens, you'll be treated with large doses of vitamin D, together with calcium supplements. Finally, as with any surgery, there is a small risk that your scar could become infected. Thyroid surgery is delicate, and it's important to have an experienced head and neck surgeon who knows what he or she is doing.

Radioactive Iodine Treatment

If you've had cancer in a secondary stage and have had a total thyroidectomy, radioactive iodine treatment will be the next step after surgery. The purpose is for "overkill"—to make absolutely certain that thyroid cancer has no chance of developing anywhere else in your body. Radioactive iodine destroys all thyroid cells and tissue in the body and therefore destroys all differentiated forms of thyroid cancer, or normal cells that could have the potential of becoming cancerous. (Chapter 10 explains radioactive iodine in detail.) You'll be given another thyroid scan to check the success of the thyroidectomy procedure, verifying how much (if any) thyroid tissue is still left in your body. Again, you are given a "tracer" of radioactive iodine (I^{123}). Usually a slightly higher dosage is required for this test. After this follow-up scan, you will probably require a "body scan," during which the imager takes pictures of your entire body to make sure the cancer has not spread beyond your thyroid.

Your doctor will take you off your thyroid replacement hormone to induce a hypothyroid state deliberately and trigger the release of thyroid stimulating hormone (TSH) into your blood. TSH will stimulate both the normal and cancerous tissue to absorb iodine, and the test becomes far more accurate. The same thing is also done when you're finally given radioactive iodine as a treatment for thyroid cancer. But there is a new way of doing a thyroid scan after a thyroidectomy that will be far more comfortable for you. Until now, the only way to measure the "success" of a thyroidectomy (after a diagnosis of thyroid cancer) was to make you hypyothyroid prior to the scan by taking you off your thyroid hormone. But a new product, known as *recombinant human thyrotropin,* will allow you to remain at normal levels for your scan. (Some studies have shown, however, that thyroid "leftover tissue" [or remnants] are more likely to be picked up by the scan using the traditional method of making you hypothyroid prior to the scan.)

Radioactive iodine treatment for thyroid cancer involves high doses. The typical dosage ranges between 100 to 150 millicuries. That's a lot. The reason for such a high dosage (anything over 30 millicuries) is that, with thyroid cancer, the aim is to kill all thyroid tissue throughout your body. It's given only as a secondary stage of treatment depending on how advanced the cancer is. It's important to note that not all thyroid experts agree about how much radioactive iodine is needed to destroy "leftover" thyroid (remnant) tissue. Some people may receive a dose as low as 29 millicuries, the maximum amount you can have without being hospitalized in North America. But all experts do agree that when all normal thyroid tissue is destroyed, it's a lot easier to detect levels of thyroglobulin in your blood (a protein made by thyroid tissue). If you're making thyroglobulin after your thyroid gland has been removed, and all the "remnant tissue" has been destroyed, it's a sign that your cancer could be recurring.

After about ten days, you may need to undergo one more scan to ensure that the treatment has *worked;* it almost always does. Once the post-treatment test has been done, you're usually home-free. Only in rare cases is treatment unsuccessful.

Radioactive Myths After talking to hundreds of thyroid patients around North America, this treatment has been the source of a huge number of myths that have a pretty long "half-life." Here are some of the most common myths I wish to dispel, once and for all.

Myth: *Radioactive iodine causes leukemia.*

Fact: Wrong! Even if you had something like 500 millicuries of radioactive iodine (Graves' disease patients can receive anything from 4 to 30 millicuries, while thyroid cancer patients get 100 to 150)—an unheard-of dosage—only about 5 of 1,000 people on that dosage would go on to develop leukemia, *which probably could not be absolutely linked to the radioactive iodine anyway.* Even given this super-exaggerated circumstance, your chances of developing leukemia are 0.5 percent.

Myth: *Radioactive iodine causes breast cancer.*

Fact: People who have undergone radioactive iodine therapy (including me) have the same chance as anyone else of developing breast cancer. Right now, we don't really know what causes breast cancer, but there is not an increased incidence of the disease in people who have received radioactive iodine. For more information on breast cancer risks, consult my book, *The Breast Sourcebook*.

Myth: *Radioactive iodine causes other kinds of cancer.*

Fact: This isn't true, either. Your chances of getting a particular kind of cancer relate to your family history and genetic makeup. This is not altered one iota by radioactive iodine.

Myth: *Radioactive iodine causes birth defects.*

Fact: This is only true if you have the treatment while you're pregnant—which would not happen, because no competent doctor in his or her right mind would ever recommend this treatment to a pregnant woman. As long as you wait six months after this treatment before trying to conceive, you'll be just fine. (Pregnancy carries other risks that have nothing to do with radioactive iodine, of course.)

Myth: *Radioactive iodine causes your hair to fall out.*

Fact. It does not. People say this because they're confusing this treatment with external radiation therapy—which also doesn't cause hair loss unless the scalp is radiated. People may also be confusing this treatment with chemotherapy, which often causes hair loss.

Myth: *People with seafood allergies cannot have radioactive iodine therapy.*

Fact: While seafood contains iodine, an allergy to seafood is rarely a reaction to iodine. People with this allergy usually do just fine. The amount of iodine in an average radioactive dose for Graves' disease amounts to less than 1 mcg anyway. But if you're concerned, see an allergist beforehand.

External Radiation

If you've had a thyroidectomy and the surrounding lymph nodes re-moved, in some instances your surgeon will want you to have radio-therapy or external radiation therapy.

During the first week of treatment, you probably won't feel much. By week two, the squared-off area that the beam targets will look like a very bad sunburn, and your throat will feel extremely sore. Swallowing will be very painful. As the treatment progresses, your throat will become so tender that you will be better off spitting out your saliva than even attempting to swallow it. You'll also feel quite tired by the third or fourth week of treatment because the procedure is mentally as well as physically draining. Be sure to discuss all poten-tial side effects of radiation therapy with your doctor before consent-ing to treatment.

Preventing Thyroid Cancer

Most of you reading this book are most likely suffering from auto-immune thyroid diseases, such as Graves' disease or Hashimoto's dis-ease, believed to be triggered, in part, by stress (see chapter 8). In these cases, there isn't much one can do to prevent thyroid disease. However, there may be ways of preventing thyroid cancer, which would prevent unnecessary suffering for thousands of people at risk due to exposure to radiactive fallout or radiation in childhood.

Potassium Iodide: A Blocking Agent

Since potassium iodide can prevent radioactive iodine from being ab-sorbed by the thyroid gland, it's known as a thyroid blocking agent. However, it can only protect against radioactive iodine; potassium iodide has no protective effect against any other kind of radiation. In fact, pharmacists report that when the Gulf War broke out, they were dispensing large quantities of potassium iodide to people who lived in communities with nuclear reactors. In some cases, doctors were prescribing it; in other cases, people were requesting potassium iodide tablets on their own.

In general, doctors are reluctant to use potassium iodide to pro-tect the thyroid unless it is "really necessary." To be effective, potassium iodide must be given just prior to someone being exposed to radioactive iodine and then continued for the duration of the exposure. This is difficult to do unless an accident is predicted in advance, or the air path of a specific accident is tracked and therefore anticipated.

Practicality is another problem; it's simply not smart to continue to administer potassium iodide over long periods of time. The main reason is because potassium iodide can have significant side effects over the long term. Complications range from a variety of serious allergic reactions, skin rashes, and thyroid disorders (such as hyperthyroidism). The thyroid problems that potassium iodide can trigger can prove particularly trying for people who have autoimmune diseases such as Graves' or Hashimoto's disease. In these cases, potassium iodide may trigger sudden hypo- or hyperthyroidism. In pregnant women, iodide can also cause the fetus to develop a goiter.

Finally, potassium iodide will have no effect as a blocking agent on people whose thyroid glands have been surgically removed or who are already taking thyroid replacement hormone tablets of some kind. In these circumstances, radioactive iodine would not be a problem because it would not be absorbed by the thyroid; the thyroid would either be gone or not functioning.

When to take it? For the last thirty years, various government agencies around the world have monitored the amount of radioactive iodine in the air. For many years, they have detected low levels of radioactive iodine fallout as a result of nuclear testing carried out across the globe (most recently by China and France). If serious nuclear reactor problems are anticipated, or occur, authorities would order the immediate distribution of potassium iodide to people who might be at risk of exposure.

In European countries, tablets are to be predistributed to households within three to six miles of nuclear plants, depending on the country. Tablets also are to be stored at central locations, such as schools, factories, and town halls, for quick distribution within 15.5 miles of plants. Anyone can buy the drug at a pharmacy without a prescription, but it is not recommended for people over age forty-five because risks may outweigh benefits. And since 1982, households within about nine miles of four nuclear plants have received tablets. Every five years, regional authorities repeat the distribution, to approximately 50,000 households, through the mail.

Distribution in the United States remains controversial. The Three Mile Island accident was the most serious reactor accident to have occurred in North America. State and federal officials are still debating potassium iodide's costs and benefits over twenty years after the nuclear accident. A presidential commission strongly recommended stockpiling the drug near all U.S. reactor sites after Three Mile Island, but the drug is now stockpiled by only Alabama, Arizona, and Tennessee. One reason is because, after Three Mile Island, it was calculated that the average population exposure from radioactive iodine in that accident was very small—much less radiation than a chest X-ray and thousands of times less than a routine diagnostic I^{131} uptake test. Because of these facts, and the possible effects of radioactive iodine, both the American and Canadian Food and Drug Administrations have not released potassium iodide as a drug for thyroid blocking, except to state/province and local governments who stockpile it for emergency use.

The information now available about the Chernobyl accident indicates that, despite the very large amounts of radioactive material that came from the Russian plant, only those working in and around the plant were exposed to any serious danger. Careful monitoring showed that no significant amounts of radioactive iodine reached North America. In the immediate vicinity of the Russian plant, Kiev, Poland, and other parts of Europe, where wind carried the fallout cloud, authorities considered the threat significant, and potassium iodide was distributed.

Thyroid Self-Exam

If you think that you have been exposed to radioactive iodine, make sure to do what I call a "Thyroid Self-Exam" or TSE, also called a Thyroid Neck Check. In fact, there is now a "Thyroid Neck Check" video, produced by the American Association of Clinical Endocrinologists, that takes you step-by-step through a "neck check." To perform a neck check, you will need a glass of water and a hand-held mirror.

1. Hold the mirror in your hand, focusing on the area of your neck just below the Adam's apple (which some people confuse with the thyroid gland) and immediately above the collarbone.
2. While focusing on this area in the mirror, tip your head back.
3. Take a drink of water and swallow.
4. As you swallow, look at your neck. Check for any bulges or a protrusion in this area when you swallow. (The thyroid gland is located further down on your neck, closer to the collarbone.)
5. Repeat this a few times to be sure that you are "all clear."

If you notice any bulges or lumps in this area, see your doctor as soon as possible to have the lump investigated.

The thyroid gland is still not at the top of the list for many specialists and primary care doctors when they are investigating vague symptoms or looking for high-risk cancers. The next chapter explains how to maximize your relationship with your primary care doctor and find a thyroid specialist. It also explains all of the tests and medications that you will encounter as you get to the bottom of your symptoms and solve that thyroid problem.

CHAPTER 10

Thyroid Doctors, Tests, and Treatments

Ask any feminist scholar about "women and doctors," and you'll get a lecture about how the medical system, designed by white men, is still in the business of *servicing* the white male body in a world designed to support white male society. There is a lot of evidence to support that claim. Much of what we know about general health is general health in a *white man's* body—because it was that body which was participating in clinical trials looking at diseases, treatments, drug interactions, and so forth. Therefore, the "norms" for a healthy body are often based on a healthy white male body—one that does not menstruate, get pregnant, breast-feed, or go through menopause. Many women die of curable diseases simply because they do not exhibit the same symptoms as men, and their symptoms are therefore missed by their doctor. Considering that women use the medical system more often than men, it is disturbing that so much information is unknown when it comes to how a given disease or drug "works" in a female body.

There is a little bit of history that many people forget when it comes to explaining why women were, until recently, excluded from clinical research trials. In the past, women, the elderly, minorities, and other vulnerable populations had a long history of being *abused* in medical research—to such an extent that public outcry demanded stronger regulations that sought to protect them. In response to the horrors of thalidomide (marketed in 1958), a "morning sickness" drug that was not properly tested prior to marketing (which caused severe limb deformities in the developing fetus), as well as DES (diethylstilbestrol—administered from the 1940s until the early 1970s), a "miscarriage prevention" drug which was later revealed to cause a rare form of vaginal cancer in "DES daughters," legislation was passed to protect pregnant women and women of childbearing potential.

The ethics of excluding women from medical research were first questioned when basic diseases, such as heart disease, were shown to manifest in completely different ways in men than in women. For example, because men suffer from heart attacks much earlier than women, heart disease suddenly became a "man's disease" even though it kills just as many women. In point of fact, women die from heart disease more than any other disease. What we know about heart disease (symptoms, prevention, treatment, etc.), therefore, is based on a man's body. As discussed in chapter 5, the symptoms of heart disease in women, and the age they "present," or manifest, are much different. But until recently, few primary care doctors were able to recognize heart disease symptoms in women. Unfortunately, the same can be said about thyroid disease.

Women also report considerable psychological and emotional abuse by male doctors or, rather, some *paternalistic* male and female doctors—doctors that behave like parents by treating adult patients like children. For example, women's health complaints are often not taken seriously. Many women are given "fluffy" answers about their symptoms, told it is "PMS" or "menopause," or sent to psychiatrists for physical symptoms.

How does this affect women with thyroid disease? Many of the doctors women will need to see when dealing with their thyroid problem will certainly be male. The message is simple: Ask questions about how X or Y affects *you*. Whether you are pregnant, going through menopause, taking hormone replacement therapy, or working a second shift, only you can individualize, and optimize, your health care.

The Right Primary Care Doctor

A primary care doctor is the doctor who you see all the time. For example, you would see this doctor for a cold, flu, or annual physical; this is the doctor who refers you to specialists.

Primary care doctors today are either *general practitioners* (four years of medical school and one year of internship), *family practitioners* (four years of medical school and a two-year residency in family medicine), or *internists* (four years of medical school and a four-year residency in internal medicine). During medical training, rotations are done in a variety of specialties such as psychiatry, endocrinology, obstetrics and gynecology, emergency medicine, and so on. During residency, the years are spent in a teaching hospital under the supervision of teaching faculty (assistant, associate, or full professors of medicine) who teach one specialty. The number of years spent in a residency program after four years of medical school varies depending on the university and the specialty. To qualify as a specialist, such as an endocrinologist, a doctor must do a residency in endocrinology. After that, a fellowship year is required, and that doctor must be eligible to write exams for the Fellowship of the American College of Physicians/Surgeons. (The letters "F.R.C.P." stand for Fellow Royal College of Physicians; "F.R.C.S." stands for Fellow Royal College of Surgeons, for physicians who received training in Canada or the U.K.) The majority of women with thyroid disease are cared for by their primary care doctors, but their quality of care may vary. What you will find today is that most primary care doctors in the U.S. become very good at treating a few conditions. Some see a lot of patients with diabetes, for example; others see more pregnant women; still others more elderly patients requiring palliative care. It all depends on the magic phrase "patient population." *Where* is the doctor's practice located? What medical plan is that doctor listed with? *Who* are the people in that neighborhood?

Therefore, a primary care physician may not be the best doctor to manage your thyroid condition if that doctor doesn't see many thyroid patients. Some doctors are also behind the times when it comes to thyroid disease and do not immediately recognize early warning signs or high-risk groups, or understand which diagnostic tests are useful and which are not. When you're diagnosed with thyroid disease, ask your doctor the following questions. They can help to determine whether you should stay with your doctor or look for another one:

1. *What is your philosophy about doing routine TSH tests (thyroid stimulating hormone level tests)?* Any doctor who does not believe a routine TSH test in women is necessary is not in step with today's medicine. Women should have their thyroid levels checked once a year, particularly those having a family history of thyroid disease, those exposed to X-ray therapy or radiation (see chapter 9), or those planning a pregnancy. Pregnant women during the first six months after delivery, and women after age fifty should, too. TSH tests are cheap, accurate, and alleviate a lot of unnecessary suffering.

2. *Will you be referring me to a specialist?* The answer should be "Yes." If you have been diagnosed with an autoimmune thyroid disease such as Graves' disease or Hashimoto's disease, you should be under the care of an endocrinologist who specializes in thyroid disease, and an opthalmologist who can monitor any eye changes (see chapter 6). If your doctor says, "I can manage your condition without referring you elsewhere," get out of that office and go elsewhere.

3. *Where can I go for more information?* Any doctor who does not refer you to one of the organizations listed in the resource (Appendix) section (see page 263) is clearly not up to date.

The Alarm Bells

If you hear the following words come out of your doctor's mouth, go elsewhere:

- "You do not need to have a TSH test; your thyroid gland is not enlarged." You do not need an enlarged thyroid gland to have symptoms of thyroid disease.
- "What is a TSH test?" Bad sign—leave immediately!

- "Radioactive iodine will give you cancer." This statement means that your doctor does not know what he or she is talking about when it comes to thyroid treatment. You should leave.
- "I don't need to check your thyroid; it's just stress." Because checking your thyroid levels are so easy to do, it is important to rule out a thyroid problem *before* you are sent to a psychiatrist or told that you're "just under stress." Stress can, in fact, trigger a thyroid problem, as discussed in chapter 8.
- "You do not need to see a specialist." (You do need to see a specialist.)

The Patient's Bill of Rights

What do you have a right to expect from a doctor?

1. *As much information as you want.* This means that you have every right to know your diagnosis, prognosis (doctor's estimate of when you will get better), alternate forms of treatment, your doctor's recommendations, and the basis of his or her recommendations (i.e., research studies, a hunch, etc.).

2. *Time to address questions and concerns.* If your doctor does not have time to answer questions, you should be able to call or make another appointment that serves as a "question and answer" session.

3. *Reasonable access.* You and your doctor must decide together what "reasonable" means. Do you need weekly, quarterly, or annual appointments? Or do you just want to see the doctor when you feel like it? How much advance time will you need to get an appointment?

4. *To participate in the decision-making process.* To do this, you will have to ask questions and be willing to educate yourself about your illness (i.e., request literature on your illness from your doctor).

5. *Adequate emergency care and to meet your doctor's substitute.* Who will look after you after hours—when your doctor is

sick or on vacation? Is there a substitute doctor? You had better find out in case you need to see the substitute one day.

6. *To know who has access to your health records.* How confidential are your health records? Can your doctor release them to just anyone—your employer, insurance companies, government authorities, etc.? What are your doctor's legal obligations with respect to health records—and what are yours?

7. *To know what it costs.* If you live in the U.S., you have the right to know what your bill is in advance. Get an estimate and have the doctor break down each charge so that you know exactly what you are paying for and what your insurance plan is covering. If you live in Canada, make sure that all appointments, tests, and procedures are covered by your province before you consent to anything.

8. *Be seen on time.* If you are on time for an appointment, your doctor should be as well. Do you generally have to wait more than thirty minutes in the reception area before your doctor will see you?

9. *To change doctors.* Yes, you can fire your doctor. If you are unhappy with your current doctor, or simply need a change, then you have every right to switch. Make sure you arrange for your records to be transferred.

10. *A second opinion, or a consult with a specialist.* If your doctor cannot make an adequate diagnosis, then you can, and should, insist on a referral to either another doctor or specialist.

The Doctor's Bill of Rights

Remember, it's a two-way street. Your doctor has an unwritten bill of rights, too. Just as you are entitled to certain information and courtesies, so is your doctor. So what exactly does your doctor have the right to expect from you?

1. *Full disclosure.* Doctors are not telepathic. If you are hiding information (certain family or medical history, prescriptions, addictions, allergies, eating disorders, specific symptoms, etc.), then it's unfair to expect an accurate

diagnosis. What if your doctor prescribes a drug that you are allergic to, for example, or one that conflicts with other medication?

2. *Common courtesy.* Treat your doctor like a business associate. If you make an appointment, show up; if you need to cancel, give at least a twenty-four-hour notice.

3. *Advance planning.* Plan your visit in advance and think carefully about your symptoms. Don't just go to your doctor with a vague complaint such as "I am not feeling well..." and expect a full diagnosis. When you make an appointment, tell the receptionist how much time you think you will need for a full examination, and write down your symptoms. Give the doctor something to work with.

4. *Questions and interruptions.* If you don't understand something, ask. Interrupt the doctor if necessary and ask for a simpler explanation of what is wrong. If you don't do this, you can't blame your doctor for not giving you enough information.

5. *Follow advice and speak up.* Take medication as directed and follow advice. That's what you are paying the doctor for. If you are experiencing side effects to medication, have a problem with the doctor's advice, or your condition has worsened as a result of the doctor's advice, let your doctor know. Full disclosure strikes again.

6. *No harassment.* If you have a problem, then use all reasonable channels; dial the after-hours emergency number that the doctor has left with the answering service, or call your doctor's office during business hours. Don't continuously call the doctor at home at 4:00 A.M., and don't call the office ten times a day to report every little ache and pain.

7. *Enough time to make a diagnosis.* Diagnoses are not arrived at overnight. Allow the doctor enough time to examine you, take necessary tests, etc. Do not expect miracles in fifteen minutes. This might mean that you need to wait longer for an appointment so that doctor can schedule enough time for a full examination.

8. *Room for disagreement.* What you think is in your best interest may not be what your doctor thinks is best. Allow for a difference of opinion and give your doctor a chance to explain his or her side. Don't just leave in a huff and threaten to sue. Maybe your doctor is right.

9. *Professional conduct.* Don't request unusual favors that compromise your doctor's moral beliefs, and don't ask your doctor to do something illegal (i.e., writing bogus notes to your employer so that you can file for disability pay).

When to Get a Second Opinion

Getting a second opinion means that you see two separate doctors about the same set of symptoms. The doctors can be in the same field or specialize in different areas. This can happen either during the diagnostic or the treatment stage of an illness. Second opinions often come into play in the diagnosis and treatment of various thyroid disorders and illnesses. Often, the doctor will want you to see one of his associates or a specialist to confirm a diagnosis or a particular treatment approach; this is known as a consult. Sometimes the patient requests a referral to another family doctor or specialist to seek an alternate diagnosis or approach to treatment; this is what we've come to know as a second opinion, although a consult is the same thing.

Second opinions can be tricky, however. First, there are a variety of factors that doctors weigh to determine the best treatment. For example, a thirty-year-old, single woman with Graves' disease may be prescribed antithyroid drugs by one doctor, while another may want to use radioactive iodine. In the first case, perhaps the doctor wishes to spare risking radioactive iodine since the woman is in her prime childbearing years; he may not want to risk radioactive iodine just in case the woman is in the very early stages of pregnancy, or he feels that the woman's anxiety over the long-term effects of the treatment may do more damage.

In the second case, the doctor may feel that radioactive iodine, a speedier and more results-oriented therapy, will treat the illness once and for all; after all, prolonging the illness will prolong the woman's suffering, and radioactive iodine is perfectly safe so long as the woman is not pregnant. Both approaches are correct, but it is the woman who will choose the treatment that she is most comfortable with. Yet the same doctor who wants to use antithyroid medication on this woman may want to use radioactive iodine on another Graves' disease patient, a woman with four children who is divorced and age forty.

On the other hand, second opinions can prove lifesaving, particularly when a thyroid disorder is misdiagnosed. For example, misdiagnosed Graves' disease symptoms are often caught by eye specialists—ophthalmologists. In these cases, patients may go to their family doctor and complain of some general hyperthyroid symptoms that imitate stress symptoms. They are told to "slow down" and come back if the symptoms persist. Not connecting their sudden eye problems to these more general symptoms, Graves' patients often seek out referrals to an ophthalmologist regarding their sudden blurred vision or pains in their eyes. At this point, it is the ophthalmologist who would diagnose exophthalmos (eye bulging), a condition caused by thyroid disease, and then refer the patient to an endocrinologist.

Or, a fifty-year-old woman with classic hyperthyroid symptoms, which include missed periods, may be diagnosed by her family doctor with menopausal symptoms and prescribed estrogen hormone supplements. (Admittedly not an outrageous diagnosis given the woman's age and symptoms.) In this case, the woman would be wise to request a referral to a hormone specialist—an endocrinologist—who would take a variety of blood tests to check her hormone levels before prescribing anything. Thyroid levels in this case would probably be routinely checked, and the woman's problem caught here.

Guidelines for Seeking a Second Opinion

It is difficult to know whether you are justified in getting a second opinion. Here are a few guidelines to help decide:

1. *Is the diagnosis uncertain?* If your doctor can't find out what's wrong, or isn't sure whether he or she is correct, then you have every right to go elsewhere.

2. *Is the diagnosis life-threatening?* In this case, hearing the same news from someone else may help you cope better with your illness, or come to terms with the diagnosis. Diagnoses like cancer, for example, usually won't change; the diagnosis is based on carefully analyzed test results—not just a patient's symptoms.

3. *Is the treatment controversial, experimental, or risky?* You might not question the diagnosis but have legitimate concerns with the recommended treatment. For example, if you are not comfortable with radioactive iodine, perhaps another doctor can recommend antithyroid drugs or surgery.

4. *Is the treatment not working?* If you are not getting better, maybe the wrong diagnosis was made or the treatment that was recommended is just not for you. Often, antithyroid medication does not work, and radioactive iodine is the best approach after all. In this case, seeing someone else may help to clear up the problem.

5. *Are risky tests or procedures being recommended?* If you don't like the sound of a radioactive iodine scan, hearing it from someone else might make you accept the procedure more readily. Or perhaps a blood test or biopsy is a better route for you. Find out if there are alternate procedures that can confirm the same results.

6. *Do you want another approach?* An eighty-year-old woman with heart disease and high blood pressure might be diagnosed with thyroid cancer. She will probably die from heart disease or a stroke before she dies from thyroid cancer, which grows very slowly. As a result, her doctor may decide that she's too frail for surgery and treatment and opt to leave her alone. The woman's children may find this approach unacceptable and demand that her thyroid cancer be treated.

7. *Is the doctor competent?* When I asked my gynecologist if radioactive iodine treatment would conflict with the Pill,

his response was: "What's radioactive iodine?" I left and never went back. I eventually found an excellent gynecologist who was well-versed in thyroid disease and cancer. Basically, if your doctor doesn't seem to know very much about your other health problems and doesn't bother to find out—go somewhere else. Or if you suspect your doctor is substandard, then go somewhere else to either reaffirm your faith or confirm your original suspicions.

Doctors Say the Darndest Things

I became convinced that this section needed to be added when I received a call recently from a young woman who had been treated for thyroid cancer. She was put on thyroid hormone replacement at too high a dosage (this happens), and she became severely hyperthyroid as a result. Her doctor's response? "You are *supposed* to be hyperthyroid after cancer treatment or else the cancer can grow back." No attempt was made to lower the dosage, perform blood tests, or even prescribe beta-blockers. When this woman phoned me, her pulse was over 200 beats per minute, and she had lost more than fifteen pounds.

"Who *is* this jerk?" I asked, wanting to know *who* could mismanage her so badly.

"It's my endocrinologist. He's the only one in town."

"Well, does this doctor treat thyroid disease or mostly diabetes?"

"Mostly diabetes."

I gave this woman the number of a thyroid foundation chapter in her area, which had lists of *thyroidologists* (a term used to describe endocrinologists who specialize in managing thyroid disease only). I told her that it was worth getting on a bus, train, or plane to have the right specialist look at her. I then explained to her that while, yes, thyroid cancer patients need to be on a higher dosage of thyroid hormone pills in order to totally suppress their TSH (I explain this below), it was absolutely not necessary for these patients to ever experience hyperthyroid symptoms. This woman and I were already buddies since her call to me the year before, when her thyroid cancer was diagnosed. In that exchange, she phoned me in tears because her family doctor said (and I quote): "I think that you're crazy for having radioactive iodine; don't you know that it causes *leukemia?*"

I yelled. What planet does he live on? I then told this woman what I say on pages 210–211 in chapter 9. (In case you missed it: radioactive iodine therapy doesn't cause leukemia, breast cancer, or any other kind of cancer.)

The point is that just because your doctor has a medical degree doesn't make them a thyroid specialist. If something doesn't sound right, it may not be. Please call either me (in care of my publisher) or any of the organizations listed at the back of this book. Don't just walk away and think, "Well, he is the doctor, so he must know best."

A dozen ways to be mismanaged Here are twelve of the most common errors primary care doctors make when misdiagnosing or mismanaging a thyroid condition:

1. Many don't know very much about radioactive iodine therapy. Therefore, a lot of misinformation and just plain *wrong* information is given to the patient. You may be told that you can never have children or that your risk of leukemia will triple. All of this is wrong, wrong, wrong. See "Radioactive Myths" in chapter 9 for more information.

2. Many will insist that you don't need to see a specialist. This is not appropriate. Many primary care doctors simply don't know. You should always have your thyroid problem assessed *first* by a specialist. Indeed, your thyroid disorder may not be complicated and may be easily managed by a primary doctor. But don't assume so until you hear firsthand from a thyroid specialist.

3. If you are lucky enough to be referred to an endocrinologist for a thyroid problem, many primary care doctors don't realize that not *all* endocrinologists are *thyroid* specialists. Many concentrate on diabetes and just "dabble" in thyroid, as referenced in the anecdote above. See "How to Find a Thyroid Specialist" on page 231 for more information.

Worse, many diabetes specialists are not aware of what they don't know about thyroid disease.

4. Many will still tell you that your symptoms are "stress-related" or "diet-related."

5. Many will ignore lumps in the neck and tell you that it is "nothing." Never ignore a lump anywhere on your body. Get a second, third, or fourth opinion if necessary before you dismiss it.

6. Many doctors will still tell you that your symptoms are related to PMS, menopause, chronic fatigue syndrome, and even chronic *yeast* of all things.

7. Many will refer you to a psychiatrist after having mistaken your symptoms for biological depression. Or you will be referred to a variety of inappropriate specialists.

8. Some will mistake Hashimoto's disease for thyroid cancer because of the firmness of the goiter. So instead of a TSH test and an antithyroid antibody test, they give you a fine needle biopsy and thyroid scan!

9. Many will fail to recognize a TSH deficiency, which means that on top of your hypothyroidism, you will experience problems with your reproductive glands (often pubic hair falls out) and adrenal glands. Symptoms range from complete loss of libido to blood sugar problems and high blood pressure. This can send you bouncing from one specialist to another for months.

10. Most will fail to distinguish between thyroid problems and aging. A classic problem is the failure to diagnose what's called "apathetic hyperthyroidism," which affects seniors. This means that you'll have slight hyperthyroidism though not severe enough to be obvious. You may have just a slight increase in your pulse rate, exhibit a slight loss of energy, and so on. Seniors represent the most underdiagnosed group of thyroid patients in the world.

11. Some doctors still prescribe thyroid hormone replacement to perfectly healthy women for weight control. Thyroid hormone replacement is not a weight-loss drug and is only

intended as treatment for hypothyroidism and other thyroid problems. A healthy person taking this medication will eventually die of heart failure. Weight problems after a thyroid problem is treated are caused by the usual suspects: lack of exercise combined with an improper diet.

12. Many primary care doctors are behind the times when it comes to thyroid testing. Thus, they order obsolete blood tests that measure bound, and hence "inactive," thyroid hormone instead of "free" and active hormone. As discussed earlier, the appropriate tests are TSH and FT4 (free T4). TT4 (total T4) is obsolete, but if it's being done, you will need to have a T3 resin uptake test as well.

How to Use a Specialist

Specialists comprise a different breed than family physicians. They're more academic: they teach or run residency programs; they're involved with research, frequently lecture at various academic centers, regularly publish papers, articles, and books in their field; and they're recognized authorities in their field. Specialists train longer than family doctors, make more money, and charge more for their services. As a result, many specialists are more egotistical, colder in terms of their bedside manner, harder to get in touch with (they're usually booked months in advance), and because they're pressed for time—impatient. Certainly there are many specialists who are very caring and do not fit this profile, but don't be surprised when you find one that is.

In addition, you usually don't have the luxury of shopping for a specialist the way you do for a family doctor because you're only referred to one when you need one. At that point, your main concern is getting better as soon as possible, and "getting in" to see another specialist can take months—time you really can't afford when you're ill.

Again, you have rights, and specialists, just like any other doctor, have their rights as well. Because their time is valuable (not to mention expensive), here are some guidelines to follow that will help you to make advantageous use of your specialist:

1. *Tape-record your visit.* Specialists often say a lot in a small space of time. When you are upset or overwhelmed by all of the information being hurled at you, you often will not fully grasp what the specialist is saying. Tape-recording the visit can prove helpful because you can replay information when you're more relaxed, and thus fully understand what you were told.

2. *Take a list of questions with you and tape-record the answers.* When you have a lot of questions, make a list so that you don't forget them. The specialist has an obligation to answer all of your questions, and if they don't have the time, there are some options. Give them your list and ask if they will address them during your next appointment. If that is not possible, then agree on a time when the specialist can call you at home and provide the answers. As a final resort, ask if there is a resident studying with the specialist with whom you can arrange a "question and answer" session. (Usually, any resident—a "specialist in training"—can address your questions.)

3. *Request literature or videos on your illness from the specialist, or the number of an organization that you can call for more information.* In my case, many of the specialists that I saw were flattered that I found "their work"—my condition— so interesting. If they have more information about your illness, they will usually be happy to share it with you.

4. *If it is relevant, ask the specialist to draw you a diagram of your illness.* My head and neck surgeon actually drew me a diagram of the thyroid, carefully explained to me where my cancer was, etc.

How to Find a Thyroid Specialist

This can be tricky, as many readers have told me. First, not all en-docrinologists handle thyroid problems. Many specialize solely in di-abetes, or even *reproductive* endocrinology. But, thankfully, many specialize solely in thyroid disorders, too. Second, if you need thyroid surgery, not all general surgeons or endocrinologists do it. And if you live in a small community where there is one endocrinologist serving the entire population (this is common; they often know more about diabetes than thyroid), then your search will be challenging. So here's the shortest route to a good thyroid specialist. (It's not foolproof, though):

1. Call a thyroid organization at the back of this book (see Appendix) for a list of thyroidologists—and use that term— in your area. If the person on the other end of the phone says, "Huh?" respond "Endocrinologists who specialize in treating thyroid disease."

2. Go to your primary doctor and ask to be referred to at least two specific names on that list (many health plans require a referral to specialists).

3. Make an appointment with *both* so you can interview them. Ask "How many thyroid cases do you manage a year?" If the answer is under ten (I am being generous), that specialist doesn't see many thyroid patients. Then ask how many diabetes patients that specialist sees per year. If the number is disproportionately higher, you may be in the wrong office. Then ask how many fertility patients that specialist sees per year (just to make sure that you didn't end up with a fertility specialist or a reproductive endocrinologist).

4. If you are still unsuccessful, ask people you know if they know someone with a thyroid problem. And then, call *them*. Who are *they* seeing? You may need to travel outside your area to a larger city. But it's worth the trip to avoid being mismanaged (which will cost you more in the long run).

5. Once you are with a thyroidologist, that doctor will manage the rest of the referrals to ophthalmologists (for thyroid eye disease); head and neck surgeons (for surgery); nuclear medicine specialists (for radioactive iodine therapy); oncologists (for thyroid cancer); etc. See the Glossary for a listing of specific terms.

What the Doctor Orders

Okay. Let's assume that you're with the right doctor! What diagnostic tests and therapies can you expect to undergo to assess and treat your thyroid condition and monitor how well you have responded to therapy?

Blood Tests

If you are suffering from hyperthyroidism, often the signs are obvious and a simple blood test called TSH test will confirm the diagnosis. TSH levels will read below normal when thyroid hormone levels are elevated. Sometimes, if a patient knows that thyroid disease runs in the family, their doctors will regularly check their thyroid function—via blood test—and can detect hyperthyroidism before any onset of blatant symptoms. But when the symptoms of hyperthyroidism are not recognized, and the patient notices only subtle differences such as irritability or fatigue, misdiagnosis can also occur.

The appropriate blood tests are those that check your *free* T4 (FT4 in labspeak) levels and your TSH. The term *free* refers to "unattached" thyroid hormone that travels in your bloodstream. Every hormone in our body tends to be "bound," or attached, to a chemical protein in our blood. The bound hormone is inactive while the free hormone is active. That's why it's crucial to measure free and, hence, active hormone. If your doctor is ordering an older test, called a "total T4" (TT4 in labspeak), this should be combined with a T3 resin uptake test, which also measures free T3. For the record, Total T4 tests are considered obsolete and have been replaced with free T4 tests. Any doctor ordering a TT4 on a blood requisition form should be asked why. To confirm or rule out an autoimmune disease such as Graves' disease or Hashimoto's disease (discussed in chapter 8), you will be tested for antithyroid antibodies or what is called thyroid stimulating antibodies.

If you are suffering from hypothyroidism, the TSH blood test can also determine low levels of thyroid hormone by rising as the result of even minimal reductions in thyroid hormone production. Another blood test can also detect the presence of antibodies in your bloodstream that point to an autoimmune disorder.

Most people feel best when their TSH readings are between 1 and 2 (the normal range is 0.5–5). A TSH of 5 or over will mean that you are probably suffering from hypothyroid symptoms, while a TSH of under 0.5 may mean that you are suffering from hyperthyroid symptoms. If you've had thyroid cancer, your TSH levels should be zero (0) to prevent a recurrence of the cancer (see page 243).

Radioactive Iodine

"Radioactive" is the adjective used to describe elements containing unstable atoms—or atoms that are emitting energy and, hence, releasing radiation. A radioactive element is called an isotope, meaning "unstable element." Radioactive iodine is used in thyroid testing, and as the standard form of treatment given exclusively to patients who are either hyperthyroid—from diseases such as Graves' disease (see chapter 8)—or who are diagnosed with thyroid cancer (see chapter 9). It is also used as a tracer for certain diagnostic tests.

The uptake test: Testing function A common test to check thyroid function is known as the "Radioactive Iodine Uptake" test. This is reserved for hyperthyroid patients only and may help to pinpoint how "abnormal" the thyroid is. (Blood tests such as the TSH test, discussed above, are still the most accurate method for determining levels of hypothyroidism.) Abnormality is determined by reading how much radioactive iodine is absorbed by the thyroid. This is a "twenty-four-hour" test.

When you arrive at the hospital that first day, you will be given a minuscule amount of radioactive iodine. It may be in the form of a capsule or water-like liquid. You ingest the iodine and go home. You are usually (but not always) given some sort of "instruction pamphlet" that tells how to reduce the risk of radiation exposure to others around you. (See below.)

There is more than one isotope or recipe of radioactive iodine available, but isotopes with an atomic weight of either 123 or 131 (usually referred to as I^{123} or I^{131}) are the ones most widely used. There is currently a debate within the nuclear medicine community as to whether I^{123} is more effective than I^{131}; some physicians believe

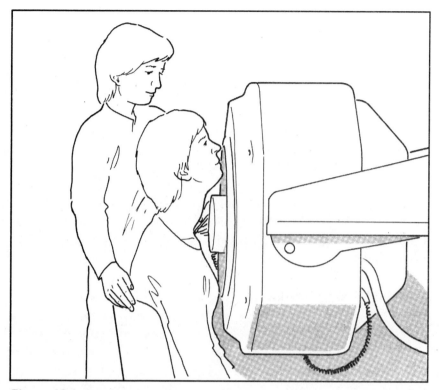

Figure 10.1 A radioactive iodine uptake test.

Reprinted from *Nichts Gutes im Schilde Krankheiten der Schiddruse.* Copyright 1994, Georg Thieme Publishing.

that I^{123} subjects patients to less radiation but does the same job as I^{131}. At any rate, the test is known as "The I^{131} Uptake Test." The next day, you return to the hospital and sit in front of a huge cameralike instrument. A cone-like device is brought right up to your neck, area and the machine then measures the amount of radioactive iodine absorbed by your thyroid by "counting" it. This instrument is known as a "scintillation," or counting probe (see Figure 10.1).

If your hyperthyroidism is caused by an overproduction of thyroid hormone, your "uptake," or absorption, of the radioactive iodine is high (usually more than 30 percent in twenty-four hours). If you are hyperthyroid but your uptake is low, your hyperthyroidism is probably caused by either an overdose of thyroid replacement hormone or some sort of inflammation in the thyroid.

If you are hypothyroid, this test is considered useless. It usually shows nothing more than a blood test would, and so it is never used.

The only time thyroid hormone readings are difficult to interpret is when you're pregnant, on oral contraceptives, or if you're taking certain medications that may interfere with thyroid hormone readings.

It's important to note that the medical philosophy/approach regarding radioactive iodine uptake tests has shifted dramatically since the early 1990s. Many endocrinologists now believe that radioactive iodine uptake tests should be reserved only to determine why you have a goiter, why you have a lump on your thyroid gland, whether you have a *cancerous* lump on your thyroid gland, and, sometimes, to determine the cause of hyperthyroidism if you test negative for Graves' disease antibodies. To order this test to simply confirm hyperthyroidism or determine "how hyperthyroid you are" is considered a waste of time and money. If your T4 readings are high and/or your TSH readings are low, you are hyperthyroid. Period.

The imaging test: Testing structure The "Thyroid Imaging Test" is similar to the Uptake Test. It is used to check thyroid structure. Also a twenty-four-hour test, the purpose of an imaging test is to check the size of a large goiter or to check for "hot" or "cold" nodes (described in chapter 9).

An imaging test is also done to check the success of a thyroidectomy procedure to verify how much (if any) thyroid tissue is still left in your body. Again, you are given a "tracer" of radioactive iodine (I^{131} or I^{123}). Usually a slightly higher dosage is required for this test. When you return to the hospital the next day, you will lie down under a large camera or imager that takes pictures of your thyroid. The iodine absorption is visible in the pictures, and your doctor can tell by the images how much structural damage is present. Sometimes a body scan is necessary if thyroid cancer is present. The only difference between a body scan and a thyroid scan is that the imager takes pictures of your entire body to ensure that the cancer hasn't spread beyond your thyroid.

If you are being given this test as a follow-up to a thyroidectomy (usually performed only in the event of thyroid cancer), your doctor will take you off your thyroid replacement hormone. This is done to deliberately induce a hypothyroid state and trigger the release of thyroid stimulating hormone (TSH) into your blood. TSH will stimulate the cancerous tissue to absorb iodine, making the test far more accurate. The same thing is also done if you are being treated for thyroid cancer.

The basic difference between an Uptake Test and an Imaging Test is that the Uptake Test measures thyroid performance, while the Imaging Test measures form.

Depending on your condition and the hospital, something called "TC pertechnotate," a more convenient tracer, is used instead of I^{131} or I^{123} for both the Uptake and Imaging tests. When TC pertechnotate is used, your thyroid is exposed to only $1/100$th of the radiation that would occur with I^{123}, for example, and the tests can be performed only twenty minutes after the tracer is administered. This is probably the new wave of radioactive iodine, and by the early twenty-first century, both I^{131} and I^{123} may very well be regarded as medical anachronisms for diagnostic testing.

Killing the Thyroid Gland

In cases such as Graves' disease, for example, radioactive iodine is used to "kill" the gland—the source of your hyperthyroidism. A by-product of this treatment may well be hypothyroidism, because once your thyroid gland is destroyed, of course, it can no longer produce thyroid hormone. It's a "feast or famine" situation. This is very easily remedied, though. Once the gland is pronounced "dead," you're immediately put on thyroid replacement hormone (to be taken daily) to bring you back to the "euthyroid," or normal state.

The treatment for Graves' disease is similar to the first stage of the diagnostic tests described earlier, only you're given a far more potent dose of radioactive iodine. A "curie" is the unit of measurement for radioactive substances. Doses of radioactive iodine are administered in either millicuries (one-thousandth of a curie) or microcuries (one-millionth of a curie).

A typical dose of radioactive iodine for treatment of Graves' disease would consist of anything between 3 to 12 millicuries, while a radioactive iodine tracer for an Uptake Test would consist of anything between 4 and 6 microcuries. A tracer for an Imaging Test (or scan) would range between 30 and 100 microcuries. A dosage over 30 millicuries requires hospitalization, but dosages for treatment of Graves' disease never reach these levels of potency. You are usually sent home immediately after treatment but must observe the rules outlined below to avoid exposing others around you to the radiation you have received.

For hyperthyroidism, usually just a single dosage is required. And it's totally painless, regardless of whether you're given a capsule or liquid. Only in very high dosages (over 30 millicuries) would you feel any discomfort. With a higher dosage you might feel some tenderness in your neck. Sometimes a high dosage affects the saliva glands and causes your mouth to feel drier after the treatment. But that's really it. You're rechecked (through a blood test, usually) at six weeks, three months, nine months, and then annually.

This brings us to one of the most misunderstood aspects of radioactive treatment. Many thyroid patients believe (a fact often reinforced by ignorant doctors) that when hypothyroidism sets in after treatment, it means you've had an "overdose" of radioactive iodine. This is just plain wrong! The point of radioactive iodine therapy is to "ablate," or destroy, the thyroid gland and turn it into something resembling a dried-up raisin. This will eliminate your hyperthyroidism permanently. So if you are *hypo*thyroid after this treatment—good! That means it worked, and you will not have to repeat the therapy. To restore thyroid hormone, all you need to do is take a pill, something I discuss at great length in the next section.

Now, some doctors enjoy the "challenge" of administering just the right amount of radioactive iodine to cure the hyperthyroidism without making you hypothyroid. This is a hotly debated issue at present. Many doctors feel this approach is fruitless due to the nature of autoimmune thyroid disease. For most cases of Graves' disease, the thyroid gland will continue to overproduce thyroid hormone no matter how "precise" a radioactive dosage you have gotten. Treatment for thyroid cancer has different goals, which are discussed in chapter 9.

It's also important to note that radioactive iodine does not go to work immediately on your hyperthyroidism. In other words, your symptoms are not going to disappear overnight. It takes at least four to six weeks, and often closer to three months, for the treatment to decrease the size of your thyroid gland as well as thyroid hormone secretion. Fifteen percent of all patients treated with radioactive iodine for hyperthyroidism will need a second dose, while 5 percent may even need a third helping. Ultimately, 20 percent of those who receive this treatment for hyperthyroidism will become hypothyroid (a sign that you are cured), and will then need to be on thyroid hormone replacement for life in order to return to a normal thyroid state. Generally, 50 percent of people treated with radioactive iodine can expect to be hypothyroid in ten years. That's why it's very important to have regular thyroid function tests every six months or so.

That said, I can't tell you how many calls I've received from readers who cry on the phone because their doctors (usually primary care physicians—who generally *do not* know a whole lot about radioactive iodine) have told them that radioactive iodine therapy can cause leukemia, breast cancer, ovarian failure, and a whole list of horrors. Any thyroid specialist will tell you that *this is just not true*. In fact, I have file folders of studies that report the same thing. Patients who have received this therapy (including me) have been followed since the 1950s and have not developed higher rates of cancer compared to the general population. If your doctor tells you otherwise, he or she is just not up on the current literature. Earlier studies suggested that one could expect 5 cases of leukemia per 1,000 patients treated with 500 millicuries of radioactive iodine—an almost unheard of amount. Essentially, stating that you're likely to develop leukemia after a standard 100 milicurie dose of radioactive iodine is as logical as saying, "Your chances of being hit by a car may increase after this therapy."

What is true, however, is that if you have had one endocrine cancer, you are statistically at increased risk for other endocrine cancers such as breast cancer. But this has *nothing* to do with radioactive iodine and everything to do with your genes and family history.

The only other risk being studied at present is the effect of radioactive iodine therapy on the salivary glands. There seems to be an increase in salivary gland inflammation (called sialoadenitis) following this therapy. Experts recommend sucking on lemons following the therapy to get your salivary glands working and stimulated.

Killing Cancer Cells

As discussed in chapter 9, radioactive iodine treatment for thyroid cancer involves a very high dosage that ranges from 100 to 150 millicuries. Again, this dosage is only given if the cancer was discovered in a secondary stage; when detected early enough, thyroid cancer can perhaps be treated through surgical means only.

After a high dose of radioactive iodine (i.e., over 30 millicuries) you are kept in isolation in a private hospital room for at least two days and not permitted any visitors. There is usually no discomfort other than the effects mentioned above with high dosages. When you are released from the hospital, you will then be required to practice the precautions listed below. After about three months you may need to undergo one more imaging test to ensure that the treatment *worked*—it almost always does—and then you are usually home-free. Only in very rare cases is treatment not successful. In these circumstances, an additional high dosage of radioactive iodine would be administered and the isolation procedures repeated.

Post-treatment precautions for regular dosage After you have received an average treatment dose of radioactive iodine, you will need to follow some hygiene precautions for the next two or three days. The reason for these precautions is to prevent the exposure of radiation to others through your saliva, sweat, mucus, urine, feces, or other bodily secretions. It's a lonely couple of days, admittedly, but it's necessary. If someone were exposed accidentally, they would not get sick, but they would be exposed to an unnecessary level of radiation that could—in a worst-case scenario—cause some harm to their healthy thyroid glands. The dosage for Graves' disease usually has a "half-life" of about eight days. That means that in eight days the radiation is half as potent as it was when it was first administered. After about two or three days, the remaining radioactive particles in your body deteriorate considerably, and you no longer pose a "threat" to anyone around you. In fact, the amount of radioactivity in your system becomes quite negligible at this point. For the first few days, the main things to keep in mind are to reduce closeness and contact with others, while keeping very clean.

You should minimize contact with pregnant women or small children because children, infants, and fetuses are more sensitive to radiation exposure. You should use different and/or disposable dishes and cutlery, and wash them separately. You should abstain from all sexual activity (including kissing), sleep alone, and wash your linens separately after use. You should use a separate hairbrush, comb, towel, and facecloth and wash out the sink or bathtub after each use. After you use the toilet you should wash your hands carefully, flush the toilet about three times per use, and use separate toilet paper. If you use the telephone, you must wipe the mouthpiece with a damp cloth after each use. You should launder separately everything you wear or use. You should also drink a lot of fluid to help pass the radioactive iodine faster through your system via your urine.

If you are a woman in your childbearing years, a pregnancy test is typically required because you *must not* be given radioactive iodine therapy if you are pregnant. The radioactive iodine can injure the thyroid gland of the developing fetus. If you are not asked to take a pregnancy test, demand one—even if you are using contraception or are menstruating regularly. It is very important that you do not take any chances. Sometimes, even after a negative pregnancy test, you can still discover that you are pregnant. (Usually, tests do not detect the pregnancy until about the sixth week.) If you have had the radioactive iodine treatment and then discover you are pregnant, your obstetrician may want to perform a "therapeutic" abortion. This really depends on the circumstances. If you are in the very early stages of pregnancy, the thyroid gland does not develop in the fetus until the twelfth week, so you are still considered safe. If you are planning to become pregnant, check with your doctor and find out how long you have to wait before you can conceive. Usually it's about six months.

If you are breast-feeding, you must stop after you have radioactive iodine because it will indeed pass through your milk to your baby. Check with your doctor to find out when you can start again. In most cases, waiting until about three months after treatment is acceptable.

When Your Doctor Tells You to Take a Pill

When you are taking thyroid medication, you are either on thyroid replacement hormone for life to compensate for a hypothyroid condition (often the result of treatment for hyperthyroidism) or you are taking antithyroid medication to control hyperthyroidism. Depending on your condition, age, sex, weight, and lifestyle habits, your doctor will recommend one of these two forms of medication.

Thyroid Hormone Replacement

In the U.S., more than fifteen million prescriptions of thyroid hormone per year are sold. Even if only part of your thyroid gland was surgically removed, thyroid hormone replacement may be prescribed.

Thyroid hormone has come a long way. In the 1890s, medical textbooks gave "recipes" for preparing animal thyroid glands as a treatment for thyroid patients. You were likely to have "fried, minced thyroid," served with bread and currant jelly for breakfast. A few decades ago, the first form of thyroid replacement hormone used was dessicated thyroid hormone, which was composed of dried animal thyroid hormone. Unlike the synthetic hormone used today, dried animal thyroid hormone was a mixture of T4 and T3, and no two mixtures of dessicated thyroid hormone were alike. For example, one pill may have contained three parts T3 and one part T4, while another contained the reverse. As a result, although dessicated thyroid hormone worked, it was jarring to other bodily systems because it was crudely produced. A prescription for thyroid hormone replacement pills costs anything from $15 to 30 for a three-month supply, depending on the brand. If you have a problem with dyes used to color the pills, most brands offer their 50 mcg strength as a plain white pill, without dye. Pharmaceutical manufacturers recommend that you ask your doctor to prescribe your thyroid hormone replacement in increments of the white pill (such as 50 mcg) if you are experiencing a reaction. See "What Is in This Stuff, Anyway?" (on page 247) for more information.

Today's thyroid replacement hormone, or synthetic thyroid hormone, comes in colored tablet form. The generic name is levothyroxine sodium. Each color represents a different strength depending on the brand. (See Table 10.1.) Thyroid hormone replacement pills are color-coded. This is done to improve what pharmacists refer to as "patient compliance." When each dosage comes in a different color, it's much easier for patients to say, "I'm taking the pink pill" than "112 mcg," for example. See Table 10.1 for a complete list of colors, dosage strengths, and suggested guidelines according to weight.

If you are taking multivitamin pills or iron supplements such as ferrous sulphate, take your thyroid hormone pill at least two hours in advance. Iron appears to bind to thyroid hormone, thus making less of it available for absorption into your body.

The right dosage If you are on too high a dosage of synthetic thyroid hormone, you will develop all of hyperthyroidism's classic symptoms. If this happens notify your doctor; your dosage will be adjusted accordingly. The correct dosage of levothyroxine sodium is determined by a normal TSH reading and other blood tests.

After treatment for hyperthyroidism, the average dose is roughly 112 mcg. Most people will be able to find the right dose for them in the seven or eight dosage strengths that various brands offer, which range from 50 to 150 mcg. The average daily dose after thyroid cancer treatment ranges from 100 to 200 mcg. Please see the next section for more information.

As discussed above, a normal TSH reading ranges from (0.5–5 mU/L). A reading greater than 5 mU/L suggests that you are hypothyroid, while a reading less than 5 mU/L suggests you are hyperthyroid. T4 readings may also be checked. The normal range is between 50 and 165 nmol/L, but most people feel best when the readings are above 110.

If you've had thyroid cancer The appropriate thyroid hormone replacement dosage is slightly different for thyroid cancer patients. That is because the goals of therapy are a little different as well. Any microscopic piece of thyroid tissue in your body will be stimulated by TSH. If that thyroid tissue is cancerous, then TSH may stimulate cancerous tissue and cause it to grow. In your case, the trick is to find a high enough dosage to suppress your TSH, which means that your

T4 readings will be *higher* than in just "plain ol' hypothyroid" patients. *But*—you need not suffer any hyperthyroid symptoms. TSH suppression can be accomplished with one of the precise doses offered by brand name thyroid hormone replacement pills. Common dosages for thyroid cancer patients are 125 or 137 micrograms (137 mcg is not available in Canada). The appropriate range for TSH suppression is anywhere from 100 to 200 mcg.

One study found that patients on thyroid hormone specifically for TSH suppression were better off waiting one hour after taking their pill in the morning before having breakfast. It was suspected that milk products had something to do with improving the absorption of the medication.

If you are elderly or have heart disease To avoid any risk of being "overreplaced" (i.e., overdosed to the point where you are hyperthyroid), dosages of thyroid hormone in your case should start fairly low, at around 12.5 mcg (a 25 mcg pill cut in half with a special pill cutter, available at all pharmacies). Dosages should be adjusted very, very slowly, in increments of 25 mcg until you reach the proper thyroid level.

What brand should I take? The key phrase in a quality thyroid hormone replacement pill is "precise dosing." This enables your doctor to prescribe the lowest, most effective dose without either overdoing it or "underdoing" it. It's also important to keep in mind that thyroid hormone brands are not interchangeable. Endocrinologists have seen as much as a fourfold difference in thyroid function after patients have switched brands. The right dose for you on Brand A may not be the right dose on Brand B.

That said, studies to date indicate no significant differences between the four most commonly dispensed brands of levothyroxine. In "clinical speak," they were found to be "bioequivalent" (absorbed in the blood in precisely the same way) and considered bioequivalent under current FDA guidelines. This means that the brands studied were found to be interchangeable in the majority of patients receiving thyroid hormone replacement therapy. But disagreement persists regarding bioequivalency among thyroid brands.

Table 10.1 The United Colors of Thyroid Hormone Replacement Pills

Thyroid hormone replacement is color-coded by dose. Dose is usually determined by weight, unless the goal is TSH suppression, or there are other medical conditions at work. Below is a *general* guideline only, in micrograms, assuming approximately 1.6 micrograms of thyroid hormone replacement daily for every kilogram of adult body weight. After age sixty-five, expect your dosage to decrease by about 10 percent. Eltroxin is available only in Canada. Levoxyl and Levothroid are available only in the United States. Please note that this table does not represent all brands of thyroid hormone sold in North America and is intended as a general guideline only.

Color	Dosage	Brands	Weight Range
orange	25	Synthroid/Levoxyl/ Levothroid	16–23 kg/30–50 lbs
white	50	Synthroid/Levoxyl/ Levothroid/Eltroxin	24–39 kg/51–87 lbs
violet	75	Synthroid	40–51 kg/88–112 lbs
purple	75	Levoxyl	SAME
gray	75	Levothroid	SAME
olive	88	Synthroid/Levoxyl	52–59 kg/113–131 lbs
mint green	88	Levothroid	SAME
yellow	100	Synthroid/Levoxyl/ Levothroid/Eltroxin	60–66 kg/132–146 lbs
rose	112	Synthroid/Levoxyl/ Levothroid	67–74 kg/147–163 lbs
brown	125	Synthroid/Levoxyl	75–86 kg/164–190 lbs
purple	125	Levothroid	SAME
dark blue	137	Levoxyl	82–91 kg/180–200 lbs
blue	137	Levothroid	SAME
light blue	150	Synthroid/Levoxyl/ Levothroid/Eltroxin	87–101 kg/191–225 lbs
lilac	175	Synthroid	SPECIAL CASES
turquoise	175	Levoxyl/Levothroid	SAME
pink	200	Synthroid/Levoxyl/ Levothroid/Eltroxin	SAME
green	300	Synthroid/Levoxyl/ Levothroid/Eltroxin	SAME

Sources: "Solving the puzzle of hypothyroidism." Physician literature, supplied by Knoll Pharma Inc., 1995; Levoxyl Prescribing Information, Daniels Pharmaceuticals, Inc., 1994; Levothroid Prescribing Information, Forest Pharmaceuticals, Inc., 1995; Eltroxin Prescribing Information, GlaxoWellcome, Inc., 1995.

For instance, one manufacturer had to recall some of its batches from the market because the batches were made from "nonmicronized" raw materials from another supplier; this meant that the drug was not being made available to the body appropriately (called bioavailability). Very simple changes in the manufacturing of levothyroxine tablets can make a big difference in performance. In addition, when the batch of thyroid pills that you receive from your pharmacist has been on the shelf for too long, the pills may not be as potent as they were when first shipped. Therefore, it's crucial to always ask when your pills *expire*. Experts also warn that a bottle of pills that expires in March 2000, which is dispensed in December 1999, should be rejected by the buyer as a batch that is not "fresh."

The shortest route to maintaining thyroid hormone function with your thyroid pill is to:

1. Choose a brand of thyroid hormone pill that offers *precise dosing*. (See Table 10.1.) This is particularly important for women over age forty who may be approaching menopause, and anyone over age sixty as well as people with heart conditions.

2. Stay on that brand; don't switch around. Again, because you may require a different dose on Brand A than you do on Brand B, just stay on your present brand.

3. Watch for signs of hyperthyroidism (see "Hyperalphabet" in chapter 2). These symptoms mean that you're on too high a dosage of thyroid hormone.

4. Watch for signs of hypothyroidism (see "Hypoalphabet" in chapter 2). These are signs that you're on too low a dosage of thyroid hormone.

5. Get a thyroid function test every three months for the first couple of years after you begin your pills; then graduate to six months; then annually.

6. Always find out when the pills expire and how long they have been on the pharmacist's shelf.

7. If you miss a pill, don't worry; just carry on the next day. Thyroid hormone pills have a very long half-life, and

missing a pill every now and then won't make any difference. If you accidentally take two pills, again, this won't make any difference. Just carry on.

8. Take your pill on an empty stomach if you can. Don't take it at the same time as a multivitamin; wait at least two hours after taking your pill before you add the multivitamin.

The Synthroid scandal The reason we know that there is no difference in bioequivalency between thyroid hormone brands is because Knoll Pharmaceutical, makers of Synthroid, initiated and funded the research that proved it. A scandal arose when Knoll decided not to publish the results of this research for seven years. In April 1997, the *Journal of the American Medical Association* published the research results anyway, while Knoll insisted that the results were kept from the public because the research was flawed, and the results were therefore invalid.

In May 1997, a class action lawsuit was filed against Knoll, claiming that thyroid patients overpaid for Synthroid during that seven-year time span by as much as three times the price of competitors' products. The lawsuit, which remains unsettled, as of this writing, demands that patients be compensated by Knoll for their overpayment.

What is in this stuff, anyway? Thyroid hormone pills contain a number of excipients (substances added to a medicine that allow it to be formed into a shape having consistency). These include diluents, lubricants, binders, and disintegrants. The pills may contain acacia, lactose, magnesium stearate, povidone, confectioner's sugar (which has corn starch), and talc. The lactose used in thyroid hormone pills is minimal; there is approximately one hundred times the amount of lactose in one-half cup of whole milk as in one tablet of Synthroid, for example. If you are highly lactose intolerant, you can take your thyroid hormone pill together with a lactose enzyme.

The T3 controversy Over the years, many readers have written to me about just not "feeling right" on their thyroid hormone pills, even though their TSH levels were normal and they were apparently taking the right dosage. An article published in the February 11, 1999, issue of the *New England Journal of Medicine* reported some dramatic findings for thyroid patients. Apparently, when the thyroid hormone with three iodine atoms (T3), known as triiodothyronine, was added to their regular thyroid hormone replacement pill (which is thyroxine, or T4, the thyroid hormone with four iodine atoms), people felt much better. A "cocktail" of T3 and T4 helped relieve depression, brain fog, fatigue, and other hypothyroid symptoms (see chapter 2). The article concluded that "treatment with thyroxine plus triiodothyronine improved the quality of life for most [hypothyroid] patients."

This may explain why some patients have felt better on alternative thyroid drugs, which contain T4 and T3 naturally (ask your pharmacist or doctor).

In any event, this comes as surprising and welcome news for many thyroid patients who thought they were suffering from phantom hypothyroid symptoms. If you are currently not feeling quite right on your thyroid hormone pill, get a copy of the article and show it to your doctor. Or photocopy this page.

Thyroid replacement hormone and other drugs Because we either combine various medications from time to time or are taking other daily medications for different health conditions, it's important to be aware of how thyroid replacement hormone medication interacts with other prescription and nonprescription drugs.

- *Oral anticoagulants (Coumadin®, Wafarin, Heparin)* An anticoagulant, or blood thinner, helps prevent blood clotting and is prescribed for a variety of heart conditions. It is also prescribed during or after surgical procedures. (Wafarin is an ingredient in rat poison, incidentally.) When combined with thyroid hormone, the anticoagulant can become more potent—which could cause minor hemorrhaging. Your doctor may need to reduce the dosage of Coumadin, Heparin, or Warfarin. This occurs only when initiating thyroxine therapy, not when patients are taking it regularly. When an elderly patient is on these drugs, their thyroid levels should be tested every six months.

- *Estrogen* This combination can increase your T4 (thyroxine) readings. It's best to get your thyroid levels checked once a year if you are taking estrogen for any reason.

- *Insulin or oral hypoglycemics* This combination lowers the effect of insulin, which means that your doctor may have to increase your insulin dosage. This occurs only when you begin taking thyroid hormone tablets. After both medications are adjusted, you should be fine. If you are diabetic, however, it's a good idea to get your thyroid levels checked once a year.

- *Anticonvulsants* Drugs such as Dilantin®, are prescribed for epilepsy; they help to prevent seizures. This combination lowers your T4 levels. It doesn't mean that you will automatically become hypothyroid, but you will probably need a lower dose and should have your thyroid levels checked about once a year.

- *Laxatives, coffee, or alcohol* Thyroxine and anything that affects the digestive system should be taken as many hours apart as possible to ensure better absorption of the thyroid medication.

- *Cholestyramine* This drug is prescribed for people with high cholesterol levels. When combined with thyroxine, this drug lowers the absorption of thyroxine. Therefore, the two should not be taken together. A space of three to four hours between each is recommended with thyroxine being taken first.

- *Antidepressants* If you are on thyroid replacement hormone and taking any one of the following antidepressant drugs: Elavil®, Asendin®, Etrafon®, Limbitrol®, Pamelor®, Surmontil®, Tofranil®, Tofranil®P.M., Triavil®, or Norpramin®, the antidepressant will become increasingly potent. This can also lead to abnormal heart rhythms. It will only happen upon beginning your thyroid medication, however, and tapers off once your medications are balanced. Be certain to get your thyroid levels checked every year, and inform whoever is managing your antidepressant medication that you are, in fact, taking thyroid hormone.

- *Lithium* Lithium is prescribed for bipolar disorder (formerly known as manic-depression). Even if your thyroid is functioning normally, lithium can cause hypothyroidism. One in ten patients on lithium will become hypothyroid: 8 to 19 percent of people on lithium become hypothyroid. Lithium has also been known to cause goiter, hyper-thyroidism, and to trigger Graves' disease. Insist that your thyroid levels are checked every six months while you're on lithium. In between, you might want to keep a log of your moods on a day-to-day basis. If you're feeling unusually depressed for long periods of time, get your thyroid levels checked—just in case.

- *Amiodarone* This is a drug used to treat atrial fibrillation, which is a heart rhythm problem. This drug contains a lot of iodine, and it's been found to induce both hypo- and hyperthyroidism; in North America, where we have sufficient iodine, hypothyroidism is more common. It's also found to accelerate Hashimoto's disease but does not cause it in people who do not suffer from it initially. Hyperthyroidism is caused by this drug if you have a toxic multinodular goiter. If you are vulnerable to thyroid disease, and you are taking this drug, request an antithyroid antibody test just in case. Since the drug is stored in body fat, it can induce a thyroid problem up to twelve months after it has been stopped.

Antithyroid Medication

The only time you will take antithyroid medication is if you are hyperthyroid. The most commonly used antithyroid drugs are Propylthiouracil (PTU) and Tapazole® (a.k.a. Methimazole). These drugs prevent the thyroid gland from manufacturing thyroid hormone, which causes the symptoms of hyperthyroid to subside. (As discussed in chapter 8, these drugs only work about 30 percent of the time.) You will probably begin to feel better within two weeks, will feel a difference by six weeks, and feel completely well again in ten to fourteen weeks. You will most likely be on antithyroid medication anywhere from six to twelve months. Your doctor will check at six months, nine months, and twelve months to see of you still need it. If your thyroid gland now functions normally, your family doctor will still check you periodically to be sure that your thyroid hormone level (T4) remains within the normal range or just above normal range.

Unlike thyroid hormone, if you forget to take a dose of antithyroid medication, you must double it on your next dose. Antithyroid medication is only potent for eight hours, so, unlike thyroid replacement hormone, if you miss a day, it matters.

Allergies Some people develop various reactions to antithyroid medications. The reactions include rashes, itching, hives, joint pains, fever, or sore throat. If this happens, stop taking the drug and call your doctor right away. Although these reactions could occur for any number of reasons that may have nothing to do with antithyroid drugs, you don't want to risk an allergy. At this point, your doctor will check your white blood cell count and make sure it's normal. If it is, your allergy symptoms have nothing to do with the antithyroid drugs and your doctor will simply resume the antithyroid medication. If your white blood cell count is decreased, then your doctor will discuss another form of treatment such as radioactive iodine therapy or surgery. Again, radioactive iodine therapy or surgery will leave you with a nonfunctioning thyroid gland that will cause you to be hypothyroid. To balance this, you'll be placed on thyroid replacement hormone.

Mothers on Tapazole or Methimazole should not breast-feed because the drug can pass to the child through the milk. However, mothers on a small dose of Propylthiouracil can still nurse because this drug does not pass into the milk *unless* the dosage is large.

Medications to Stay Away from While You Are Hyperthyroid

- Avoid cough/cold medicines with decongestants. These drugs can cause restlessness, while stimulating your heart. Because your heart is already being overstimulated by your hyperthyroid condition, you don't want to tempt fate and risk any added stimulation. (However, mild exercise and sexual activity are fine!)

- Avoid other stimulants such as caffeine (coffee, chocolate, etc.), alcohol, or tobacco. Again, these stimulants will increase your heart rate.

- Avoid anything with excess iodine. Some prescription and over-the-counter drugs contain iodine such as certain asthma medications, vitamin pills, cough medicines, suntan lotions, and salt substitutes. Be sure to read labels before taking any other medications while you're hyperthyroid. You should also stay away from kelp (seaweed) and cut down on seafood while you're hyperthyroid. The iodine in these substances can make your hyperthyroidism worse by triggering the thyroid gland to make more thyroxine with the extra iodine.

- Do not take Haldol® if you're hyperthyroid. Haldol is a drug prescribed for certain psychiatric disorders (it is an antipsychotic) and is also widely used to control alcohol withdrawal by recovering alcoholics. Hyperthyroid patients taking Haldol may develop extreme stiffness or rigidity which could lead to an inability to walk.

- If you have been prescribed beta-blockers to control your heart rate and are asthmatic, some can trigger asthma attacks. Be sure to consult with your doctor or pharmacist about your asthma before going on beta-blockers.

Know your thyroid history and make sure to communicate your thyroid legacy to your children. That way, potential thyroid patients will know who they are and be conscious of obvious thyroid disease symptoms as they age. Their doctors will also be alerted to the possibility of a future thyroid disorder.

Whether you're reading this page as a mere browser or as someone who just finished reading the entire book, the best thing that you can do to help educate the public about thyroid disease is to pass on what you know to other thyroid patients and doctors. Recommend books, such as this one, articles, or pamphlets that you come across about thyroid disease. And don't be afraid to ask questions or start conversations with "I read that . . . "

Good luck and good health.

Glossary

Note: This list is not exhaustive. These are not literal (dictionary) definitions; rather, they have been crafted solely to fit the context of this book. Any resemblance to definitions found in other glossaries or dictionaries is purely coincidental.

Achropachy: A condition characterized by swollen fingertips.

Acute suppurative thyroiditis: A rare condition usually observed in children where a pus-forming bacterial infection develops on the thyroid gland.

Addison's disease: Occurs when your adrenal glands fail to make cortisone and steroid hormones—the adrenal products that the body requires to function properly.

Adenoma: Involves glandular cells that usually clump together in a harmless, benign lump. Since the thyroid is a gland, any benign tumor that develops on the thyroid is called an adenoma.

Amenorrhea: Absence of a menstrual cycle.

Androgenic side effects: Appearance-related side effects such as weight gain and acne.

Anemia: Occurs when there is a decrease in the number of red blood cells carrying oxygen to various body tissues. A more serious type of anemia, called pernicious anemia, is caused by a deficiency of vitamin B_{12}, and tends to occur in older people who either have, or have had, Graves' disease or Hashimoto's disease.

Anesthesiologist: A physician who specializes in administering anesthetic prior to or during surgery.

Anorexia nervosa: An eating disorder characterized by a refusal to eat.

Antibodies: Produced by the body, they attack foreign intruders called antigens. Antibodies are made from one type of white blood cell (called lymphocytes), and each antibody is designed to combat a specific virus.

Anticoagulant: A blood thinning drug that helps to prevent clotting and is prescribed for a variety of heart conditions. May also be employed/used during or after surgical procedures.

Anticonvulsants: Drugs that help to prevent seizures.

Antithyroid drugs: Drugs that prevent the thyroid from manufacturing thyroid hormone.

Atrial fibrillation: A common heart rhythm abnormality characterized by a slight pause of the heart, followed by bursts of pounding, rapid heartbeats.

Autoantibodies: Specific antibodies that attack specific organs developed by a body suffering from an autoimmune disorder.

Autoimmune disorder: Occurs when your body loses the ability to distinguish foreign tissue from normal tissue. It confuses the two and perceives healthy organs as invading viruses. Your body then begins attacking its own organs.

Bipolar disorder: Formerly called manic-depression, this is a psychiatric disease where people experience extreme mood swings from euphoria to depression. Bipolar disorder is caused by an imbalance in brain chemistry and can be controlled by taking lithium, which can cause hypothyroidism.

Bulimia: An eating disorder characterized by cycles of bingeing and purging.

Calcitonin: A hormone produced in the thyroid gland by nonthyroid cells called C cells. This hormone helps to regulate calcium.

Carcinoma: Refers to a malignant (cancerous) growth that involves the epithelial cells, which line the surface of our insides. When a tumor in a glandular area is malignant and stems from these epithelial cells, it is referred to as an adenocarcinoma.

Carotene: A substance in our diet that is normally converted to vitamin A. This is a process that slows down due to hypothyroidism.

Carpal tunnel syndrome: A repetitive strain injury characterized by tingling and numbness in the hands. Occurs when increased fluid in your wrists cuts off the nerve in the wrist responsible for feeling in the fingers and hands. In the case of hypothyroidism, this condition is caused by compression on nerves in the wrist due to water retention and bloating.

Cold nodule: A lump on the thyroid gland comprised of more primitive cells.

Combination OCs: Oral contraceptives containing both estrogen and progestin.

Congenital: A term meaning "present at birth."

Congenital hypothyroidism: Occurs when a baby is born with no thyroid gland.

Core needle biopsy (or cutting needle biopsy): Similar to fine needle aspiration (FNA), this procedure is done if FNA is not available. It requires the use of a local anesthetic.

Cretinism: Unnatural physical stunting and mental retardation caused by severe hypothyroidism.

Curie: The unit of measurement for radioactive substances.

Depo-Provera: A contraceptive that works by injection of time-released progesterone.

Dilation and curretage (D&C): A procedure using a spoon-like instrument to scrape out the lining of the uterus.

Dilation and evacuation (D&E): This is a procedure that can be performed at any point in the second trimester. A D&E is almost identical to a first trimester abortion.

Diplopia: Double vision.

Dyslexia: A correctable learning disability characterized by delays in physical or speech development, poor spelling or handwriting, stuttering, right-left confusion, and reversal of numbers or letters.

Edema: Water retention.

Endocrinologist: A doctor who specializes in glands and hormones (the endocrine system). A hormone specialist.

Endometriosis: A disease affecting women in their reproductive years. Characterized by an abnormal growth of endometrial tissue.

Endometrium: The lining of the uterus that shelters a fertilized egg and secretes embryo-nourishing substances. This is what sheds during menstruation.

Euthyroid: A term used to describe normal levels of thyroid function (*eu* means "normal").

Excipients: Substances added to a medicine that allow it to be formed into a shape and consistency.

Exophthalmometer: An instrument that measures the degree to which the eyes have become bulgy.

Exophthalmos: Bulging, watery eyes characteristic of patients suffering from thyroid eye disease (TED).

Fallopian tubes: These tubes connect the ovaries to the uterus.

Fetal thyrotoxicosis: Occurs when maternal thyroid-stimulating antibodies cross the placenta, as in the case of Graves' disease, causing the fetus to be hyperthyroid.

Fine needle aspiration (FNA): A diagnostic procedure using a needle to suck out cells and/or fluid (fluid if it is a cyst), which is sent off to a pathologist who is then able to determine if the lump is benign or malignant.

Follicle stimulating hormone (FSH): Released by the pituitary gland, this hormone stimulates the growth of the follicles containing the eggs which, as they grow, produce the hormone estrogen.

Gastroenterologist: A G.I., or gastrointestinal specialist.

GnRH (gonadotrophin-releasing hormone): Activated by the hypothalamus, this hormone stimulates the pituitary gland to release FSH.

Goiter: An enlarged thyroid gland which can develop when you produce too much thyroid hormone or too little. If your thyroid gland absorbs too much iodine, it can produce either too little or too much thyroid hormone.

Goiter belt: A term referring to regions where people typically suffer from insufficient iodine. This can cause goiters.

Graves' disease: Occurs when the body produces a thyroid stimulating antibody (TSA) that stimulates the thyroid gland to overproduce thyroid hormone in vast quantities. The result is hyperthyroidism.

Gynecologist: A doctor who specializes in caring for a woman's reproductive organs as well as her breasts.

Hashimoto's disease: A disease where abnormal blood antibodies and white blood cells attack and damage thyroid cells causing inflammation of the thyroid gland and subsequent hypothyroidism.

Hashitoxicosis: A "combo platter" of hyperthyroidism and hypothyroidism experienced by some people with Hashimoto's disease.

Hot nodule: A lump on the thyroid gland comprised of functioning thyroid cells.

Hyperthyroidism: Occurs if your thyroid gland manufactures too much thyroid hormone (hyper means "too much"). Sometimes called an overactive thyroid producing "speedy" symptoms (see the "Hyperalphabet Soup" section in chapter 2).

Hypothyroidism: Occurs if your thyroid gland manufactures too little thyroid hormone (hypo means "too little"). Sometimes called an underactive thyroid that produces "slowing down" symptoms (see the "Hypoalphabet Soup" section in chapter 2).

Hysterectomy: Surgical removal of the uterus.

Immunosuppressed: A term that describes a person susceptible to opportunistic infections (that would otherwise be harmless).

Inflammatory bowel disease (IBS): An umbrella term that comprises Crohn's disease as well as colitis. IBS is a miserable condition where the lower intestine becomes inflamed, causing abdominal cramping, pain, fever, and mucusy, bloody diarrhea.

Interstitial cystitis: Found in many women with chronic cystitis, interstitial cystitis is an inflammation of the interstitium, the space between the bladder lining and bladder muscle.

Intrauterine device (IUD): A tiny contraceptive device that fits inside the uterus.

Lobectomy (or partial thyroidectomy): Surgical removal of only part of the thyroid gland.

Lupus: An autoimmune condition that affects many body tissues causing arthritic symptoms, skin rashes, kidney, lung, and heart problems.

Luteinizing hormone (LH): Released by the pituitary gland when estrogen levels are high. When LH peaks, you ovulate.

Lymph nodes: Located throughout the body, their purpose is to capture unwanted viruses or foreign cells that continuously invade our system, and destroy them.

Mania: Euphoric mood witnessed in bipolar disorder (formerly called manic-depression).

Medullary thyroid cancer: A rare, inherited thyroid cancer characterized by an oversecretion of calcitonin. (See calcitonin.)

Megabecquerel: The term now coming into use as a unit of measurement for radioactive substances.

Metastasis: This term means "invasion," and often refers to active, abnormal cells that mass produce and invade, or metastasize, to other parts of the body.

Multinodular goiter: When bumps or lumps form on the thyroid gland that may mimic the gland in every conceivable way, which can interfere with normal thyroid function.

Myasthenia gravis: A rare autoimmune disorder of the muscles that is ten times more common in Graves' disease patients.

Myxedema: A condition characterized by thickening of the skin and underlying tissues.

Needle biopsy: A diagnostic test involving the insertion of a needle into the thyroid gland in order to remove some of its cells for purposes of examination.

Neonatal: A term referring to the first twenty-eight days of life after birth.

Nontoxic multinodular goiters: Multinodular goiters that do not cause hyperthyroidism.

Norplant: A subdermal implant and contraceptive device.

Obstetrician: A doctor who specializes in prenatal care and delivery.

Oncologist: A cancer specialist.

Onycholysis: A condition characterized by partial separation of the fingernails from the fingertips.

Ophthalmologist: An eye specialist.

Osteoblasts: The cells responsible for building bone.

Osteoclasts: Cells that remove old bone so that the new bone can be replaced.

Osteoporosis: Literally means "porous bones," a condition common to post-menopausal women.

Ovaries: Part of the female reproductive system. The ovaries make both eggs and hormones.

Palliative: A form of treatment that targets the symptoms rather than the disease.

Parathyroid glands: Everyone has at least four of these glands, located on the back of each lobe of your thyroid gland. They control calcium levels.

Pelvic inflammatory disease (PID): Occurs when an STD remains undiagnosed and invades the pelvic region, damaging the reproductive organs.

Phytoestrogens: These are plant estrogens said to be therapeutically beneficial for symptoms of menopause.

PID (pelvic inflammatory disease): A chronic condition that refers to infection and inflammation of the pelvic organs.

Pituitary gland: Also called the master gland, the pituitary gland keeps track of your age, begins your reproductive cycle at puberty, controls your body during pregnancy, and ends your cycle at menopause. It is situated at the base of the skull. The thyroid gland reports directly to it.

Platelet disorders: Common in people with either hyper- or hypothyroidism, these disorders occur if the number of your platelets—which help your blood to clot—are reduced.

Polycystic ovary syndrome: A condition that can affect fertility. Occurs when your ovaries have small cysts that interfere with ovulation and hormone production.

Postpartum hypothyroidism: Experienced by 5 to 18 percent of new mothers. Results when the thyroid gland becomes inflamed after delivery and hypothyroidism results. Often misdiagnosed as postpartum depression.

Postpartum thyroid disease: When thyroid disease develops after delivery.

Potassium iodide: A thyroid blocking agent which can prevent radioactive iodine from being absorbed by the thyroid gland.

Premenstrual syndrome (PMS): A real biochemical hormonal condition preceding menstruation that causes both physical and emotional symptoms.

Progesterone: Often referred to as the "pregnancy hormone," this is the hormone responsible for preparing the lining of the uterus for pregnancy.

Progestin: Synthetic progesterone.

Prolactin: The hormone responsible for milk production.

Radioactive: The adjective used to describe elements containing unstable atoms or elements that are emitting energy and hence releasing radiation. A radioactive element is called an isotope, meaning "unstable element."

Radioactive iodine: Iodine in radioactive form used in the testing and treatment of various thyroid conditions.

Radioactive iodine uptake test: An imaging test that involves a tiny dose of radioactive iodine as a tracer. This test determines why you have a goiter, why you have a lump on your thyroid gland, whether you have a cancerous lump on your thyroid gland, and sometimes can determine the cause of hyperthyroidism if you test negative for Graves' disease.

Radiologist: A doctor who specializes in reading imaging tests.

Radiotherapist: A doctor who specializes in radiation therapy.

Reflux: Occurs when semidigested food comes back up the esophagus.

Rheumatoid arthritis: A disease that can cause inflammation of many joints in the body including knuckles, wrists, and elbows.

Riedel's thyroiditis: The rarest form of thyroiditis, this condition occurs when the thyroid gland is somehow replaced by a kind of scar tissue. The term *ligneous* (meaning "woody") or fibrous (meaning "scar tissue") is used to describe this peculiar condition.

Scintillation: Also called a counting probe, this machine measures the amount of radioactive iodine absorbed in your thyroid by "counting" it.

Silent thyroiditis: Similar to subacute thyroiditis, this infection causes no symptoms or outward signs of inflammation but can result in mild hyperthyroidism.

Solitary toxic adenoma: Occurs when a clump of cells or a singular growth develops and takes over all thyroid gland function. The adenoma is toxic in this case because it causes hyperthyroidism.

Subacute viral thyroiditis: Also known as de Quervain's thyroiditis, this is a condition imitating the flu, which is probably caused by one or more viruses. As the illness progresses, your thyroid gland will swell and become very tender, sometimes resulting in hyperthyroidism.

Subclinical hypothyroidism: Refers to hypothyroidism that has not progressed very far and is still asymptomatic.

Synthetic thyroid hormone: Prescribed as a supplement when treating hypothyroidism or prescribed as a replacement hormone when the thyroid is either removed surgically or deadened by radioactive iodine.

Thyroglobulin: A specific protein made only by your thyroid gland. It is used mostly by the thyroid gland itself to make thyroid hormone.

Thyroid gland: A butterfly-shaped gland located in the lower part of your neck in front of your windpipe, this gland produces thyroid hormone, one of the basic regulators of every cell and every tissue within the body.

Thyroid scan: An imaging test that photographs the structure of the thyroid gland.

Thyroidectomy: Surgical removal of the thyroid gland.

Thyroiditis: Inflammation of the thyroid gland.

Thyroidologist: An endocrinologist subspecializing in thyroid disease.

Thyrotoxic: Literally meaning "thyroid toxic."

Thyroxine: One of two hormones produced by the thyroid gland. Thyroxine is also known as T4 (four iodine atoms).

Triiodothyronine: Also known as T3 (three iodine atoms), triiodothyronine is the second of two hormones produced by the thyroid gland.

TSA (thyroid simulating antibody): An armed antibody produced by the body in cases of Graves' disease. TSA is sent on a special search and destroy mission and launches a surprise attack on your thyroid gland.

TSH (thyroid stimulating hormone): A stimulating hormone secreted by the pituitary gland when thyroid hormone levels are low. A TSH test is a blood test that checks your TSH levels. Low levels mean that you are hyperthyroid; high levels mean that you are hypothyroid.

Urethra: A tube that connects the bladder to the outside.

Uterus: The uterus, or womb, is more of a vessel or receptacle (for the fetus) than an organ and is controlled entirely by hormones.

Vitiligo: A skin condition that results in patches of pigmentation loss.

Where to Go for More Information

Note: Because of the volatile nature of many health and nonprofit organizations, some of the addresses and phone numbers below may have changed since this list was compiled.

General Information

American Foundation of Thyroid Patients
  Please send your request for information and physician referrals along with a self-addressed #10 envelope with $2 for postage and handling to:
  P.O. Box 820195, Houston, TX 77282-0195
  (281) 496-4460 • Fax: (281) 496-0369
  www.thyroidfoundation.org
  E-mail: thyroid@flash.net
Thyroid Foundation of America, Inc.
  40 Parkman Street, Boston, MA 02114-2698
  1-888-996-4460
  www.tfaweb.org/pub/tfa
  E-mail: tfa@clark.net
Thyroid Foundation of Canada
  1040 Gardiners Road, Suite C, Kingston, Ontario, Canada, K7P 1R7
  1-800-267-8822
  http://hom.ican.net/~thyroid/canada.html
  E-mail: thyroid@limestone.kosone.com
Thyroid Society for Education and Research
  7515 South Main Street, Suite 545, Houston, TX 77030
  1-800-THYROID
  www.the-thyroid-society.org
  E-mail: help@ the-thyroid-society.org

Autoimmune Disorders

American Autoimmune Related Diseases Association, Inc.
  Michigan National Bank Bldg.
  14475 Gratiot Avenue, Detroit, MI 48205
  (313) 371-8600 • Fax: (313) 372-1512

National Association for Rare Disorders (NORD)
  P.O. Box 8923, New Fairfield, CT 06812-1783
  1-800-999-NORD

Congenital Hypothyroidism

CHAPS (Congenital Hypothyroidism and Parents' Support Group)
  8 Rockhill Court, Edwardsville, IL 62025
  (618) 692-1761

Directories

The American Board of Medical Specialties
  1 Rotary Center, Evanston, IL 60201

American Medical Association
  Division of Survey and Data Resources
  515 North State Street, Chicago, IL 60610

Marquis Who's Who
  Macmillian Directory Division
  3002 Glenview Road, Wilmette, IL 60091

Graves' Disease

National Graves' Disease Foundation
  2 Tsitsi Court, Brevard, NC 28712
  (704) 877-5251 or send SASE with your information request
  www.ngdf.org
  E-mail: ngdf@citcom.net

Nederlandse Vereniging van Graves Patenten
  Heemskerk Klein Elsbroek 3, 2182 TE Hillegom
  The Netherlands

Hair Loss

American Hair Loss Council
  1-800-274-8717

Buyer's Guide to Wigs and Hairpieces:
  Write to Ruth L. Weintraub
  420 Madison Avenue, Suite 406, New York, NY 10017
  (212) 838-1333

Edith Imre Foundation for Loss of Hair
    30 West 57th Street, New York, NY 10019
    (212) 757-8160 • Wig Hotline: (212) 765-8397

Iodine Deficiency Disorders (IDD)

International Council for Control of Iodine Deficiency Disorders (ICCIDD)
    J. T. Dunn, M.D.
    Box 511, University of Virginia Medical Center
    Charlottesville, VA 22908

Nuclear Medicine
    Society of Nuclear Medicine
    475 Park Avenue South, New York, NY 10016
    (212) 889-0717

Thyroid Eye Disease

Thyroid Eye Disease Association
    34 Fore Street, Chudleigh, Devon, U.K. TQ13 0HX
    Phone/fax: 44-1626-852980
    http://home.ican.net/~thyroid/international/TED.html

Thyroid Federation International

Associazione Italiana Basedowiani e Tiroidei (Italy)

Australian Thyroid Foundation (Australia)

National Graves' Disease Foundation (U.S.A.)

Schilddrusen Liga (Germany)

SCHILDKLIERSTICHTING Nederland (The Netherlands)

Thyreoidea Landsforeningen (Denmark)

Thyroid Eye Disease Association (U.K.)

Thyroid Foundation of America, Inc. (U.S.A.)

The Thyroid Foundation of Canada (Canada)

Vastsvenska Patientforeningen for Skoldkortelsjoka (Sweden)

Thyroid Specialists

American Association of Clinical Endocrinologists
    2589 Park Street, Jacksonville, FL 32204-4554
    (904) 384-9490 • Fax: (904) 384-8124

American Thyroid Association, Inc.
    Montefiore Medical Center
    111 East 210th Street, Bronx, NY 10467
    (718) 882-6047 • Fax: (718) 882-6085
    Physician referral: 1-800-542-6687

The Endocrine Society
 4350 East West Highway, Suite 500, Bethesda, MD 20814-4410
 (301) 941-0200 • Fax: (301) 941-0259

Other Websites:

EndocrineWeb: www.endocrineweb.com

Mining Company Guide to Thyroid Disease: http://thyroid.miningco.com

Women's Health Resources
General Gynecological Health

American Medical Women's Association (AMWA)
 801 North Fairfax, Suite 400, Alexandria, VA 22314
 (703) 838-0500
 www.amwa-doc.org

Center for Medical Consumers and Health Care Information
 237 Thompson Street, New York, NY 10012
 (212) 674-7105
 www.medicalconsumers.org

Concord Feminist Health Centre
 38 South Main Street, Concord, NH 03301
 (603) 225-2739

Lyon-Martin Women's Health Services
 1748 Market Street, Suite 201, San Francisco, CA 94102
 (415) 565-7667

Women's Health Information Center
 Boston Women's Health Book Collective
 47 Nichols Avenue, Watertown, MA 02172
 (617) 974-0271
 E-mail: office@bwhbc.org
 www.ourbodiesourselves.org

Hysterectomies

Hysterectomy Educational Resources and Services (HERS)
 422 Bryn Mawr Avenue, Bala Cynwyd, PA 19004
 (215) 667-7757

Infertility

Adopted Families of America
 2309 Como Avenue, St. Paul, MN 55108
 (612) 535-4829

Compassionate Friends
    P.O. Box 1347, Oak Brook, IL 60521
    (Provides support after miscarriage or death of a child.)

Concerned United Birthparents (CUB)
    2000 Walker Street, Des Moines, IA 50317

Fertility Research Foundation
    877 Park Avenue, New York, NY 10021
    (212) 744-5500
    E-mail: frsbabymsn.com

North American Council on Adoptable Children
    970 Raymond Avenue, Suite 106, St. Paul MN 55114-1149
    (651) 644-3036
    E-mail: nacac@aol.com
    www.members.aol.com/nacac

Pregnancy and Infant Loss Centre
    1421 East Wayzata Boulevard, #70, Wayzata, MN 55391
    (612) 473-9372

Resolve, Inc.
    1310 Broadway, Somerville, MA 02144
    (617) 623-0744
    www.resolve.org

Menopause

American Association of Retired Persons (AARP)
    Program Department
    601 E Street NW, Washington, DC 20049
    (202) 434-2277
    www.aarp.org

American Health Care Association
    1201 L Street NW, Washington, DC 20005
    (202) 842-4444
    www.ahaca.org

National Women's Health Network
    514 10th Street NW, Washington, DC 20004
    (202) 347-1140

North American Menopause Society (NAMS)
    P.O. Box 94527, Cleveland, OH 44101
    (216) 844-8748
    E-mail: info@menopause.org
    www.menopause.org

Menstruation
Society for Menstrual Cycle Research (SMCR)
10559 North 104th Place, Scottsdale, AZ 85258
(602) 451-9731

Osteoporosis
National Osteoporosis Foundation
1150 17th Street NW, Suite 500, Washington, DC 20036
(202) 223-2226
www.nof.org

Pregnancy and Childbirth
American Academy of Husband-Coached Childbirth (AAHCC)
P.O. Box 5224, Sherman Oaks, CA 91413
(818) 788-6662

American College of Obstetricians and Gynecologists
409 12th Street, Washington, DC 20024
(202) 638-5577
www.acog.org

American Gynecological and Obstetrical Society
c/o James R. Scott, M.D.
University of Utah
50 North Medical Drive, Salt Lake City, UT 84132
(801) 581-5501

Healthy Mothers, Healthy Babies
121 North Washington Street, Suite 300, Alexandria, VA 22314
(703) 836-6110
www.hmhb.org

Informed Homebirth Inc.
P.O. Box 3675, Ann Arbor, MI 48106
(734) 662-6857

International Childbirth Education Associates (ICEA)
P.O. Box 20048, Minneapolis, MN 55420
(612) 854-8660
www.icea.org

National Association of Childbearing Centers (NACC)
3123 Gottschall Road, Perkiomenville, PA 18074
(215) 234-8068
E-mail: REACHNACC@birthcenters.org
www.birthcenters.org

Bibliography

"The AACE Thyroid Neck Check." Posted online at: http://www.aace.com/ pub/spec/tam98/card.html (February 2, 1999).

"Antibiotics in Animals: An Interview with Stephen Sundlof, D.V.M., Ph.D." International Food Information Council, 1997.

"The Antioxidant Connection: Visiting Speakers Discuss Immunity, Diabetes." Published by the Vitamin Information Program of Hoffman-La Roche Ltd., September 1995.

"Are All Nodules Cancerous?" Patient education brochure. The Thyroid Society for Education and Research, 1992.

"Armour Thyroid—Company E-mail Contact for Information." Posted online at: http://thyroid.miningco.com/librar...kly/aa120998.htm?pid=2750&cob =home (February 8, 1999).

"Autoimmune Thyroid Diseases." *Thyroid Signpost* 1, no. 5 (August 1993).

Beardall, Ross A. "Thyroid Disease in Pets." *Thyrobulletin* 16, no. 2 (summer 1995).

Becker, David. "Radiation and the Thyroid." *Thyrobulletin* 16, no. 3 (autumn 1995).

Benvenga, Salvatore et al. "Delayed Intestinal Absorption of Levothyroixine." *Thyroid* 5, no. 4 (August 1995).

Bequaert Holmes, Helen. "A Call to Heal Medicine." *Feminist Perspectives in Medical Ethics* (Indiana University Press, 1992).

Berndl, Leslie. "Understanding Fat." *Diabetes Dialogue* 42, no. 1 (spring 1995).

"Blood Test Detects Thyroid Cancer Gene," *Thyrobulletin* 16 (spring 1995).

Bogdanova, Tatyana I., and Nikolaj D. Tranko. "The Dynamics of Thyroid Cancer in Children in Ukraine After the Chernobyl Accident." Institute of Endocrinology and Metabolism, Academy of Medical Sciences of Ukraine, Kyiv, Ukraine. n.d.

Bogner, U. et al. "Association Between Thyroid Cytotoxic Antibodies and Atrophic Thyroiditis." *Clinical Thyroidology* 8, no. 1 (January–April 1995).

"British Researcher Indicates That High Normal-Range TSH Values May Be 'Significant Departure from Normal.'" Posted online at: http://www.bmj.com/cgi/content/full/314/7088/1175 (April 19, 1997).

Brody, Jane E. "Tears—There May Not Be Enough." *New York Times,* December 23, 1997.

Bunevicius, Robertas et al. "Effects of Thyroxine as Compared with Thyroxine plus Triiodothyronine in Patients with Hypothyroidism." *New England Journal of Medicine* 340, no. 6 (February 11, 1999).

Cass, Hyla. *St. John's Wort: Nature's Blues Buster.* (New York: Avery Publishing Group, 1998).

Chesler, Phyllis. *Women and Madness* (New York: Avon Books, 1972).

"Cholesterol and Thyroid Disease." *Thyroid Signpost* 1, no. 2 (May 1993).

Clark, Orlo H., and Johann Elmhed. "Thyroid Surgery—Past, Present, and Future." *Thyroid Today* 8, no. 1 (March 1995).

"Combat Job Stress: Does Work Make You Sick?" Posted online at: http://www.convoke.com/markjr/cjstress.html (February 12, 1999).

Cooper, David S. "Thyroid Nodules and Thyroid Cancer: Evaluation and Treatment." *Thyrobulletin* 16, no. 3 (autumn 1995).

Costin, Carolyn. *The Eating Disorder Sourcebook* (Los Angeles: Lowell House, 1996).

"Countries That Use Nuke Pill." Posted online at: http://dailynews.yahoo.com/headlines/ap/science/story.html?s=v/a.../nuclear_pill_glance_1.htm (March 17, 1999).

Dadd, Debra Lynn. *The Nontoxic Home and Office* (Los Angeles: Jeremy P. Tarcher, 1992).

Daniels, Gilbert H. "Graves' Eye Disease." *Thyrobulletin* 15, no. 4 (January 1995).

Davies, Terry F. "New Thinking on the Immunology of Graves' Disease." *Thyroid Today* 15, no. 4 (1992).

Delange, F. "Iodine Deficiency Disorders and Their Prevention: A Worldwide Problem." Abstract from the 6th International Thyroid Symposium, Thyroid and Trace Elements, 1996.

"Depression and Thyroid Disease." *Thyroid Signpost* 1, no. 3 (June 1993).

"Depression Medicines Can Kill Women's Sex Drive." *The Vancouver Sun,* May 5, 1997.

Dirusso, G. et al. "Complications of I–131 Radioablation for Well-Differentiated Thyroid Cancer." *Clinical Thyroidology* 8 (January–April 1995).

Dong, B. J. et al. "Bioequivalence of Generic and Brand-Name Levothyroxine Products in the Treatment of Hypothyroidism." *Journal of the American Medical Association* 277, no. 15 (April 16, 1997): 1199–200.

Dottorini, M. E. et al. "Effect of Radioiodine for Thyroid Cancer on Carcinogenesis and Female Fertility." *Clinical Thyroidology* 8, no. 1 (January–April 16, 1997): April 1995).

Dreher, Henry, and Alice D. Domar. *Healing Mind, Healthy Woman* (New York: Henry Holt and Company, 1996).

Emanuel, Ezekiel J., and Linda L. Emanuel. "Four Models of the Physician-Patient Relationship." *Journal of the American Medical Association* 267, no. 16 (1992): 2221–26.

"Endocrinology and Thyroid Disorders." Posted online at: http://www.endo-society.org/pubaffai/factshee/thyroid.html (February 2, 1999).

Engel, June V. "Beyond Vitamins: Phytochemicals to Help Fight Disease." *Health News* 14 (June 1996).

———. "Eating Fiber." *Diabetes Dialogue* 44, no. 1 (spring 1997).

Eskin, B. A. "Effects of Iodine Therapy on Breast Cancer and the Thyroid." Abstract from the 6th International Thyroid Symposium, Thyroid and Trace Elements, 1996.

"The Facts About Thyroid Nodules." Patient education brochure. Daniels Pharmaceuticals, Inc., 1995.

"FDA Approves Sibutramine to Treat Obesity." FDA Talk Paper, Food and Drug Administration, U.S. Department of Health and Human Services, 1997.

Findlay, Deborah, and Leslia Miller. "Medical Power and Women's Bodies," in B. S. Bolaria and R. Bolaria, eds. *Women, Medicine and Health* (Halifax, Nova Scotia: Fernwood Books, 1994).

Fransen, Jenny, and I. Jon Russell. *The Fibromyalgia Help Book* (St. Paul Minn.: Smith House Press, 1996.)

Fraser, Elizabeth, and Bill Clarke. "Loafing Around." *Diabetes Dialogue* 44, no. 1 (spring 1997).

Gaitan, Eduardo "Goiter." *The Bridge* 10, no. 3 (fall 1995).

Garton, M. et al. "Effect of L-Thyroxine Replacement on Bone Mineral Density and Metabolism in Premenopausal Women." *Clinical Thyroidology* 8, no. 1 (January–April 1995).

Gaz, Randall D. "Instructions for Patients Undergoing Thyroid Needle Biopsy." *Thyrobulletin* 14, no. 4 (autumn 1993).

"Getting to the Roots of a Vegetarian Diet." Vegetarian Resource Group 1997.

Gilligan, Carol. *In a Different Voice.* 2d ed. (Boston: Harvard University Press, 1993).

Ginsberg, Jody. "Wilson's Syndrome and T3." *Thyrobulletin* 15, no. 4 (January 1995).

Glinoer, D. "The Thyroid Gland and Pregnancy: Iodine Restriction and Goitrogenesis Revealed." *Thyroid International* 5 (1994).

Gomez, Joan. *Coping with Thyroid Problems* (London: Sheldon Press, 1998).

"Graves' Eye Disease." *Thyroid Signpost* 1, no. 6 (September 1993).

Greenberg, Brigitte. "Stress Hormone Linked to High-Fat Snacking in Women." *The Associated Press,* April 4, 1998.

Greenspan, Miriam. *A New Approach to Women and Therapy,* 2nd ed. (BlueRidge Summit, Penn.: Tab Books, 1993).

"Hair Loss and Thyroid Disease." *Thyroid Signpost* 1, no. 1 (April 1993).

"Hanford Downwinders Can Get Radiation Dose Estimates." Posted online at: http://thyroid.miningco.com/librar...kly/aa120998.htm?pid=2750&cob =home (February 8, 1999).

Hart, Ian R. "Does Your Patient Have a Thyroid Problem?" *Medicine North America* (February 1996).

Havas, S., and J. M. Hershman. "Action of Lithium on the Thyroid." Abstract from the 6th International Thyroid Symposium, Thyroid and Trace Elements, 1996.

"Heart Disease and Stroke." Patient education brochure. The Heart and Stroke Foundation of Ontario, 1997.

"The Heart Healthy Kitchen," in *Countdown USA: Countdown to a Healthy Heart.* Allegheny General Hospital and Voluntary Hospitals of America, Inc., 1990.

Hetzel, Basil, S. "Iodine Deficiency and Excess: A World Problem." *Thyrobulletin* 16, no. 3 (autumn 1995).

"High-Carbohydrate Diet Not for Everyone." *Reuters,* April 16, 1997.

Ho, Marian. "Learning Your ABCs, Part Two." *Diabetes Dialogue* 43, no. 3 (fall 1996).

Hoffman, David L. "Hyperthyroidism." Posted online at: http://www.healthy.net/hwlibrarybooks/hoffman/immune/hyperthy-roid.htm (February 2, 1999).

Horn-Ross, P. L. et al. "Rationale for a Study of Iodine, Selenium and Thyroid Cancer." Abstract from the 6th International Thyroid Symposium, Thyroid and Trace Elements, 1996.

"How Do I Choose a Healthy Diet?" Patient education brochure. The Heart and Stroke Foundation of Ontario, 1997.

"How to Deal with Stress." Posted online at: http://www.backrelief.com/ stress.htm (February 12, 1999).

Hunter, J. E., and T. H. Applewhite. "Reassessment of Trans Fatty Acid Availability in the U.S. Diet." *American Journal of Clinical Nutrition* 54 (1991): 363–69.

Hurley, Jane, and Stephen Schmidt. "Going with the Grain." *Nutrition Action* 10–11 (October 1994).

"IFIC Review: Uses and Nutritional Impact of Fat Reduction Ingredients." International Food Information Council, 1995.

"Iodine Deficiency on Rise in U.S." *Journal of Clinical Endocrinology and Metabolism* 88 (October 8, 1998): 3401–8.

Ito, Masahiro et al. "Childhood Thyroid Diseases Around Chernobyl Evaluated by Ultrasound Examination and Fine Needle Aspiration Cytology." *Thyroid* 5, no. 5, (1995).

Jamison, Kay Redfield. *An Unquiet Mind: A Memoir of Moods and Madness* (New York: Vintage Books, 1995).

Joffe, Russell, and Anthony Levitt. *Conquering Depression* (Hamilton, Ontario: Empowering Press, 1998).

Khatamee, M. D. "Infertility: A Preventable Epidemic?" *International Journal of Fertility* 33, no. 4 (1988): 246–51.

Kotulak, Ronald. "Researchers: Lack of sleep may cause aging, stress, flab." *Chicago Tribune* (April 5, 1998).

Kra, Siegfried J. *What Every Woman Must Know About Heart Disease* (New York: Warner Books, 1996).

Kushi, Mishio. *The Cancer Prevention Guide* (New York: St. Martin's Press, 1993).

Lark, Susan M. *Chronic Fatigue and Tiredness* (Los Altos, Calif.: Westchester Publishing Co., 1993).

Leibenluft, Ellen. "Why are so may women depressed?" *Women's Health* 9, no. 2 (summer, 1998).

Leshin, Len. "The Thyroid and Down Syndrome." Posted online at: http://www.ds-health.com/thyroid.htm (April 12, 1999).

Leutwyler, Kristin. "Dying to be Thin." *Women's Health* 9, no. 2 (summer, 1998).

Levine, R. J. *Ethics and Regulation of Clinical Research* (New Haven: Yale University Press, 1988).

Lichtenstein, A. H. et al. "Hydrogenation Impairs the Hypolipidemic Effect of Corn Oil in Humans." *Arteriosclerosis and Thrombosis* 13 (1993): 154–61.

Linton, Marilyn. *Taking Charge by Taking Care* (Toronto: Macmillan Canada, 1996).

Loebig, Poertl et al. "Regulation of Maternal Thyroid During Pregnancy by Human Chorionic Gonadotropin (hCG)." Abstract from the 6th International Thyroid Symposium, Thyroid and Trace Elements, 1996.

"Major Causes of Ill Health." *Rachel's Environment & Health Weekly* #584. Posted online by the Environmental Research Foundation (February 2, 1998).

"Major Exposé on Illnesses Surrounding Nuclear Facilities." Posted online at: www.tennessean.com/special/oakridge/part3/frame.shtml (February 8, 1999).

"The Many Aspects of Subclinical Hypothyroidism." Physician literature. Toronto: Knoll Pharma Inc., 1995.

"The Many Faces of Undiagnosed Hypothyroidism." Physician literature. Toronto: Knoll Pharma Inc., 1995.

Martino, E. et al. "Increased Susceptibility to Hypothyroidism Inpatients with Autoimmune Thyroid Disease Treated with Amiodarone." *Clinical Thyroidology* 8, no. 1 (January–April 1995).

Mastroianni, Anna C., Ruth Faden, and Daniel Federman, eds. *Women and Health Research: Ethical and Legal Issues of Including Women in Clinical Studies,* vol. 1 (Washington, D.C.: National Academy Press, 1994).

Matoo, T. K. "Primary Hypothyroidism Ecodary to Nephrotic Syndrome in Infancy." *Clinical Thyroidology* 8, no. 1 (January–April 1995).

Mitchell, Marvin L. "Congenital Hypothyroidism." *The Bridge* 10, no. 4 (winter 1995).

Myers, Michael. "Sibutramine: A Medication to Assist with Weight Management." Posted online at: http://www.weight.com/sibutramine.html (July 18, 1999).

Nelson, Philip K. "Defining Chronic Fatigue Syndrome." *The Manasota Palmetto,* January 1995.

"Nutrition News." *Diabetes Dialogue* 43, no. 4 (winter 1996).

"Nutrition News." *Diabetes Dialogue* 44, no. 1 (spring 1997).

Nygaard, B. et al. "Acute Effects of Radioiodine Therapy on Thyroid Gland Size and Function in Patients with Multinodular Goiter." *Clinical Thyroidology* 8, no. 1 (January–April 1995).

"Oats Are In." *Countdown USA: Countdown to a Healthy Heart.* Allegheny General Hospital and Voluntary Hospitals of America, Inc., 1990.

"Olestra: Yes or No?" *Diabetes Dialogue* 43, no. 3 (fall 1996)

Olveira, G. et al. "Altered Bioavailability Due to Changes in the Formulation of a Commercial Preparation of Levothyroxine in Patients with Differentiated Thyroid Carcinoma." *Clinical Endocrinology* 46 (June 1997): 707–11.

Orbach, Susie. *Fat Is a Feminist Issue* (New York: Berkley Books, 1990).

O'Riordain, D. S. et al. "Impact of Biochemical Screening of Medullary Thyroid Cancer: Extent of Disease and Outcome in Patients with Multiple Endocrine Neoplasia." *Clinical Thyroidology* 8, no. 1 (January–April 1995).

Palmer, Gabrielle. *The Politics of Breastfeeding* (London: Pandora Press, 1993).

"Part 3—Treatments for Hyperthyroidism." Posted online at: http://thyroid.miningco.com/library/weekly/aa030998.htm (March 9, 1998).

Pellegrino, Edmund D., and D. C. Thomasma. "The Good Physician" in *For The Patient's Good* (New York: Oxford University Press, 1998).

Perros, P. et al. "Natural History of Thyroid Associated Ophtalmopathy." *Clinical Thyroidology* 8, no. 1 (January–April 1995).

"Proper Knowledge of a Healthy Diet Makes Huge Difference." *The Globe and Mail,* November 1, 1996.

Purdy, Laura M. *Reproducing Persons: Issues in Feminist Bioethics* (Ithaca: Cornell University Press, 1996).

"Putting Fun Back into Food." International Food Information Council, 1997.

"Q & A about Fatty Acids and Dietary Fats" International Food Information Council, 1977.

Quinn, Brian P. *The Depression Sourcebook* (Los Angeles: Lowell House, 1997).

"Recap of First Thyroid Cancer Conference Online." Posted online at: http://thyroid.miningco.com/library/weekly/aa110298.htm (February 8, 1999).

Recer, Paul. "Women Hurt More, in More Places, but Cope Better, Studies Say." *The Associated Press,* April 7, 1998.

Reiners, Chr. "Radioactive Iodine and the Risk of Thyroid Cancer." Abstract from the 6th International Thyroid Symposium, Thyroid and Trace Elements, 1996.

"Research Finds Most Patients Feel Better with Addition of T3, Not Levothyroxine (i.e., Synthroid) Alone!!!" Posted online at: http://thyroid.miningco.com/library/weekly/aa021199.htm?pid=2750&cob=home (February 11, 1999).

"The Return of Sunny Spring Isn't the Cure for All Cases of Seasonal Depression. Sometimes It Is the Cause." Posted online by Deborah Franklin, *Health Magazine* (1996).

Robinson, Melissa B. "Officials Mull Anti-Radiation Pill." Posted online at: http://dailynews.yahoo.com/headlines/ap/washington/story.html?s=v/ap/1.../nuclear_pill_1.htm (March 17, 1999).

———. "Potassium Iodide Stirs Controversy." Posted online at: http://dailynews.yahoo.com/headlines/ap/science/story.html?s=v/ap/1999.../nuclear_pill_1.htm (March 17, 1999).

Rosen, Irving B., and Paul Walfish. "You and Thyroid Cancer," *Thyrobulletin* 16, no. 4 (January 1996).

Rosenthal, M. Sara. *The Breastfeeding Sourcebook,* 2nd ed. (Los Angeles: Lowell House, 1999).

———. *The Breast Sourcebook* (Los Angeles: Lowell House, 1996).

———. *The Breast Sourcebook,* 2nd ed. (Los Angeles: Lowell House, 1999).

———. *The Fertility Sourcebook* (Los Angeles: Lowell House, 1996).

———. *The Fertility Sourcebook,* 3rd ed. (Los Angeles: Lowell House, 1999).

———. *The Gastrointessinal Sourcebook* (Los Angeles: Lowell House, 1999).

———. *The Gynecological Sourcebook* (Los Angeles: Lowell House, 1995).

———. *The Gynecological Sourcebook,* 3rd ed. (Los Angeles: Lowell House, 1999).

———. *The Pregnancy Sourcebook,* 3rd ed. (Los Angeles: Lowell House, 1999).

———. *The Thyroid Sourcebook,* 1st ed. (Los Angeles: Lowell House, 1993).

———. *The Thyroid Sourcebook,* 2nd ed. (Los Angeles: Lowell House, 1996).

———. *The Thyroid Sourcebook*, 3rd ed. (Los Angeles: Lowell House, 1998).

———. *The Type 2 Diabetic Woman* (Los Angeles: Lowell House, 1999).

Ross, Douglas S. "Fine Needle Aspiration Biopsy of Thyroid Nodules." *Thyrobulletin* 14, no. 4 (autumn 1993).

"Screening for Thyroid Cancer." Posted online at: http://cpmenet.columbia. edu/texts/gcps/gcps0028.html (February 10, 1999).

"Seaweed Snackers Risk Iodine Overdose." Posted online at: http://thyroid. miningco.com/librar...kly/aa120998.htm?pid=2750&cob=home (February 8, 1999).

Sherwin, Susan. *Patient No Longer: Feminist Ethics and Health Care* (Philadelphia: Temple University Press, 1984).

"Sibutramine: Replacement for "Fen/Phen?" Medical Sciences Bulletin, No. 239. Posted online at: http://pharminfo.com/pubs/msb/ sibutramine239.html (September 7, 1997).

Singer, Peter A. "Hashimoto's Thyroiditis." *Thyrobulletin* 16, no. 1 (spring 1995).

Singh, A. et al. "Thyroid Antibodies as a Predictor of Early Reproductive Failure." *Clinical Thyroidology* 8, no. 1 (January–April 1995).

Sloca, Paul. "After 14 Years, Nuclear Fallout Study Leads to Questions, Few Answers." *Associated Press*, August 15, 1997. Posted online at: http:// www.stardem.com.

"Smoking Affects Graves' Disease Treatment." Posted online at: http:// thyroid. miningco.com/librar...kly/aa120998.htm?pid=2750&cob=home (February 8, 1999).

Solomon, Diane. "Fine Needle Aspiration of the Thyroid: An Update." *Thyroid Today* 16, no. 3 (September 1993).

"Solving the Puzzle of Thyroid Therapy." Physician literature. Toronto: Knoll Pharma, Inc. 1995.

"Some Reasons for the Rise in Work Stress." Posted online at: http:// www.convoke.com/markjr/streesb.html (February 12, 1999).

"Sorting Out the Facts About Fat." International Food Information Council, 1997.

"Stress." Posted online at: http://meagherlab.tamu.edu/M-Meagher/ Abnormal/stressout.html (February 12, 1999).

"Study Further Links Smoking to Depression." *Reuters News Service*, February 10, 1998.

Surks, Martin I. *The Thyroid Book* (Yonkers: Consumer Reports Books, 1994).

"Synthroid Under Siege." Posted online at: http://thyroid.miningco.com/li- brary/weekly/aa022499.htm?pid=2750&cob=home (February 24, 1999).

"TED (Thyroid Eye Disease)." Patient education brochure. Lea House, Deven, United Kingdom, 1995.

"10 Tips to Healthy Eating" American Dietetic Association and National Center for Nutrition and Dietetics, Toronto, April 1994.

"Thyroid Cancer." Posted online at: http://endocrineweb.com/ thyroidca.html (February 8, 1999).

"Thyroid Cancer." Posted online at: http://www.medicinenet.com/Script/ Main/Art.asp?li=MNI&ag=Y&ArticleKey=495 (February 4, 1999).

"Thyroid Cancer: Papillary Cancer... The Most Common Thyroid Cancer." Posted online at: http://endocrineweb.com/capap.html (February 8, 1999).

"Thyroid Disease and Osteoporosis." Patient education brochure. British Thyroid Foundation and the National Osteoporosis Society, 1992.

"Thyroid Disease and Sexual Dysfunction." Posted online at: http://thyroid.miningco.com/library/weekly/aa030899.htm?pid=2750&cob=home (March 8, 1999).

"To Confirm the Clinical Diagnosis." Patient education brochure. British Thyroid Foundation, 1992.

Toft, Anthony D. "Other Forms of Hyperthyroidism." *Thyrobulletin* 16 no. 3 (autumn 1995).

"Treatment Options for Hyperthyroidism and Graves' Disease." *Thyroid Signpost* 1, no. 4 (July 1993).

Tuttle, R. Michael, Troy Patience, and Steven Budd. "Treatment with Propylthiouracil Before Radioactive Iodine Therapy is Associated with a Higher Treatment Failure Rate Than Therapy with Radioactive Iodine Alone in Graves' Disease." *Thyroid* 5, no. 4 (August 1995).

Utiger, Robert D. "Follow-Up of Patients with Thyroid Carcinoma." *The New England Journal of Medicine* 337, no. 13 (September 25, 1997).

Van Middlesworth, L. "Usual and Unusual Isotopes in the Thyroid." Abstract from the 6th International Thyroid Symposium, Thyroid and Trace Elements, 1996.

Varl, B., J. Drinovec, and M. Bagar-Posve. "Iodine Supply with Mineral Water." Abstract from the 6th International Thyroid Symposium, Thyroid and Trace Elements, 1996.

Walfish, Paul. "Thyroid Disease During and After Pregnancy." *Thyrobulletin* 16, no. 3 (autumn 1995).

"Warning Signs." Posted online at: http://home1.pacific.net.sg/choco/ tws.htm (February 4, 1999).

Wesche, M.F. et al. "Long-Term Effect of Radioiodine Therapy on Goiter Size in Patients with Nontoxic Multinodular Goiter." *Clinical Thyroidology* 8, no. 1 (January–April 1995).

Westcott, Patsy. *Thyroid Problems: A Practical Guide to Symptoms and Treatment* (London: Thorsons/HarperCollins, 1995).

"What About Tests and Treatment?" Patient education brochure. The Thyroid Society for Education and Research, 1992.

"What Is Graves' Eye Disease?" Posted online at: http://www.the-thyroid-society.org/faq/35.html (February 8, 1999).

"What Is Hyperthyroidism?" Patient education brochure. The Thyroid Society for Education and Research, 1992.

"What Is Hypothyroidism?" Patient education brochure. The Thyroid Society for Education and Research, 1992.

"What Is Thyroid Disease?" Patient education brochure. The Thyroid Society for Education and Research, 1992.

"What Is Thyroiditis?" Patient education brochure. The Thyroid Society for Education and Research, 1992.

"Who Is Likely to Become Hyperthyroid?" Posted online at: http://www.synthroid.com/thyroid_d...ent_education/hyperthyroidism.html (February 8, 1999).

Willett, W. C. et al. "Intake of Trans Fatty Acids and Risk of Coronary Heart Disease Among Women." *Lancet* 341 (1993): 581–85.

"Women Find Themselves Courted by Pharmaceutical Firms." *The Associated Press,* July 20, 1998.

Wood, Lawrence C. et al. "Your Thyroid: A Home Reference," 3rd ed. (New York: Ballantine Books, 1995).

"Your Medical Test Guide." *Health for Women* 8, no. 2 (spring/summer 1998).

"Your Thyroid." Posted online at: http://endocrineweb.com/thyroidca.html (February 8, 1999).

Zellerbach, Merla. *The Allergy Sourcebook* (Los Angeles: Lowell House, 1995).

Zimmerman, Mary K. "The Women's Health Movement: A Critique of Medical Enterprise and the Position of Women," in M. Farle and B. Hess, eds., *Analysing Gender* (Thousand Oaks, Calif.: Sage, 1987).

Index